I-Can't-Chew Cookbook

Praise for the first edition, the best-selling *Non-Chew Cookbook*

"Nearly 200 spiral-bound pages of liquid and soft-food recipes for denture-wearers, people recovering from jaw or throat surgery, and some cancer patients. All recipes have nutrient information."

— Good Housekeeping

"What he developed not only helped his wife but drew a response from thousands of desperate people across the country"

— Tampa Tribune

"The book features caloric intake tables, a food groups table and a helpful hints section to get through this period of life."

— St. Louis Globe-Democrat

"They're easy, tasty dishes with a wide range of meats, fruits and vegetables. Wilson has earned an impressive list of endorsements for his books."

— Detroit Free Press

"No-chew recipes with more punch than strained carrots and runny mashed potatoes. Wilson not only is thoughtful, he is also ingenious."

— The Phoenix Gazette

"A creative new cookbook should be a welcome wonderland of fresh ideas. If you love fine food but can't prepare or chew most recipes, order the *Non-Chew Cookbook*."

— The Miami Herald

"The number of orders for the book is clear evidence that many people crave such suggestions and recipes for tasty foods."

— The Orlando Sentinel

◇ ◇ ◇

"For millions of people who have lost their chewing functions—even temporarily—because of facial skeleton malformations, dentures, cancer of the mouth, TMJ disorders, minor oral surgery, [this book] may just put the bite back into eating."

— *Dentistry Today*

"Innovative, appetizing recipes for a group of people with serious eating problems. The book is helpful and practical."

— *Richard S. Rivlin, M.D., Chief of Nutrition, Memorial Sloan-Kettering Cancer Center*

"The *I-Can't-Chew Cookbook* is well organized, easy to read, and very appealing. I admire the systematic way Randy Wilson has gone about putting the book together. It is truly needed, and I look forward to using it for many years to come."

— *Peter E. Dawson, D.D.S., St. Petersburg, Florida*

"This masterful treasury of nutritionally sound and appetizing recipes stemmed from Mr. Wilson's loving need to help his wife. I feel this book offers exceptional variety to soft-food dieters."

— *K. Eric Alpha, D.D.S., M.S.D., Grand Junction, Colorado*

"The *I-Can't-Chew Cookbook* impressed me because it caters to a segment of the population that has been completely ignored to date. The recipes can be used by everyone in the family, not just the individual with the swallowing or chewing disorder. Nutritious and appetizing recipes everyone would enjoy!"

— *Jennifer Anderson, M.S., R.D., Food and Nutrition Extension Specialist, Colorado State University*

◇ ◇ ◇

"The ramifications of the *I-Can't-Chew Cookbook* are enormous. It is a must-read for all who are unable to chew due to TMJ dysfunction, dental problems, or other health restrictions. It gives a comprehensive and detailed nutritional analysis of the recipes. The *I-Can't-Chew Cookbook* is a much needed resource in developing and maintaining a nutritional diet, which is so essential for healing and well-being."

— *Diane K. Hartley, R.P.T., St. Petersburg, Florida*

"It fills a much needed niche for total patient care. Patients find the recipes tasty as well as nutritionally sound."

— *Barry Staley, D.D.S., Aptos, California*

"Thank you for allowing me to preview the *I-Can't-Chew Cookbook*. I believe the book will prove to be of great value to a large number of patients who are unable to chew because of ailments of the mouth and teeth, and you have performed a considerable service to these people in writing it."

— *Dhadrasain Vikram, M.D., Memorial Sloan-Kettering Cancer Center, New York, New York*

If you would like more information on this subject,
e-mail the author at randyw94@mymtnhome.com.

Ordering

Trade bookstores in the U.S. and Canada please contact
Publishers Group West
1700 Fourth Street, Berkeley CA 94710
Phone: (800) 788-3123   Fax: (800) 351-5073

For bulk orders please contact
Special Sales
Hunter House Inc., PO Box 2914, Alameda CA 94501-0914
Phone: (510) 899-5041   Fax: (510) 865-4295
E-mail: sales@hunterhouse.com

Individuals can order our books by calling **(800) 266-5592**
or from our website at **www.hunterhouse.com**

I-Can't-Chew
Cookbook

Delicious Soft-Diet Recipes for
People with Chewing, Swallowing
and Dry-Mouth Disorders

J. Randy Wilson

Foreword by Mark A. Piper, DMD, M.D.

Hunter House Inc., Publishers
PO Box 2914
Alameda CA 94501-0914

Library of Congress Cataloging-in-Publication Data

Wilson, J. Randy.
    I-can't-chew cookbook : delicious soft-diet recipes for people with chewing, swallowing and dry-mouth disorders / J. Randy Wilson ; foreword by Mark A. Piper.
        p. cm.
Includes index.
ISBN-13: 978-0-89793-400-8 (pbk. : alk. paper)
ISBN-13: 978-0-89793-399-5 (cloth : alk. paper)
ISBN-13: 978-0-89793-593-7 (ebook)
    1. Deglutition disorders—Diet therapy—Recipes. I. Title.
RC815.2 .W556 2003
616.3'10654—dc21   2002151930

Project Credits

Cover Design: Peri Poloni and Jinni Fontana
Book Design and Production: Jinni Fontana Graphic Design
Copy Editor: Kelley Blewster
Recipe Editors: Sue Spitler and Pat Molden
Nutrition Consultant: Linda Yoakam, M.S., R.D., L.D.
Proofreader: John David Marion
Acquisitions Editor: Jeanne Brondino
Editor: Alexandra Mummery
Editorial Assistant: Caroline Knapp
Publicity Coordinator: Lisa E. Lee
Sales & Marketing Coordinator: Jo Anne Retzlaff
Customer Service Manager: Christina Sverdrup
Order Fulfillment: Lakdhon Lama
Administrator: Theresa Nelson
Computer Support: Peter Eichelberger
Publisher: Kiran S. Rana

Manufactured in the United States of America

11 10 9 8 7   Second Edition   13 14 15 16 17

Contents

Foreword

The greatest pleasure that a cookbook can offer is a palatable selection of appetizers, soups, vegetables, entrées, and desserts that fulfill our need for gustatory enjoyment. The *I-Can't-Chew Cookbook* certainly meets that requirement. However, the primary motivation behind this book is to offer nutritionally balanced and tasteful recipes to individuals whose choice of foods is limited by their inability to chew.

Millions of Americans suffer from the consequences of poor chewing function. For many, this has been the result of birth deformity, and for others it has been secondary to facial trauma or surgical alteration. Given the limitation of abnormal mastication, these individuals find little to rejoice about in most cookbooks.

The number of people in the United States with loss of chewing function is enormous. Malformations of the facial skeleton, with significant alteration in the structures of the bite complex, occur in approximately five out of every one hundred births. More serious facial deformities and clefts of the facial bones occur in one out of every six hundred births. These individuals, if their problems are left uncorrected surgically and orthodontically, face a lifetime of nutritional compromise because of their inability to chew common foods. Their attempts at proper dietary intake may be a difficult, if not impossible, task to undertake.

Edentulous people, that is, those who've lost their teeth, form the largest group with permanent compromise in chewing ability. Twenty-five million Americans have lost their teeth due to dental caries and periodontal disease. The more fortunate ones are fitted with prosthetic teeth that offer an adequate replacement for their lost natural ones. The remainder, however, either cannot be fitted with dentures or cannot afford the reconstructive surgery and dentistry available to rebuild the mouth structures. When faced with the loss of a function that was once enjoyed daily, and perhaps taken for granted, these people not only lose the ability to eat certain foods, but also may deprive themselves of the will to gain adequate nutrition because of psychological depression associated with the lost ability to chew.

Another major nutritional public-health problem is found in persons with malignancies. Cancer of the mouth is discovered each year in sixty thousand Americans. Care of this dreadful menace may force the surgeon to remove major structures of the mouth, facial skeleton, or neck. Heroic reconstruction techniques may restore normal appearance for a fraction of these individuals. However, whether they undergo reconstruction or not, their ability to chew is reduced, and if nutrition is not maintained, life expectancy can be further compromised.

Other groups also bear the burden of decreased chewing function. Headache sufferers, such as Randy Wilson's wife, may endure years of chronic headache and facial pain secondary to bite problems and disorders of the temporomandibular joints. This debilitating pain, found 90 percent of the time in young females, may be misdiagnosed for years as migraines, tension headaches, or premenstrual syndrome. The frustration faced by many of these individuals as they seek aid from one physician after another eventually leads to a resolution to live with the pain. If left undiagnosed, most temporomandibular joint (TMJ) patients will discover that much of their headache pain relates directly to the chewing of coarse food. For those who are fortuitous enough to be diagnosed, the specialist may prescribe a soft or "nonchewing" diet as part of the correction of the problem.

Tens of millions of other Americans suffer temporary loss of mastication each year. This may be the result of minor oral surgery, reconstructive jaw surgery, or infections of the mouth. The serious consequences of acquired malnutrition are usually not seen in this group of patients. However, adequate nutritional intake to ensure proper healing is a necessity, even when chewing is limited for only a few days.

Most cookbooks emphasize the taste of the food. When the person with altered chewing function consults such a cookbook, he or she is disappointed with the variety of foods available to him or her.

The good food that most of us take for granted has become for him or her a burden to chew or swallow. Selections may become narrowed to those items that are easiest to eat or most convenient. As the variety of foods decreases, necessary nutrients are no longer attained, and proper nutrition suffers. This in turn may lead to the consequences of malnutrition and undernutrition, including disability, disease, poor healing, and mental anguish.

Because of a decrease in food choices, individuals on a liquid or soft diet must have a basic understanding of nutrition. Proper nutrition should supply adequate calories, minerals, vitamins, water, and fiber. Protein, carbohydrates, and fat provide the calories necessary for the energy requirements of the body. Depending upon a person's sex, body build, surgical status, and activity level, greater or less caloric intake may be required. Minerals and vitamins provide no calories, but they are essential in maintaining the metabolic processes of the body. Minerals are important components of body tissues, blood, iron, and bone. Both minerals and vitamins function in the utilization of energy and in the building and healing of body tissues. Water makes up about 70 percent of the total body weight, and it is important in the absorption of nutrients and the elimination of waste products.

In determining how we can best balance calories, vitamins, and minerals, nutritional allowances have been developed by the Food and Nutrition Board of the Institute of Medicine, part of the National Academy of Sciences. The Food and Nutrition Board has formulated Dietary Reference Intakes (formerly called Recommended Dietary Allowances) to guide daily nutrient intake for maintenance of good nutrition for the general population of the United States. A table of these recommended dietary allowances is included in Chapter 2, "More Nutritional Information." These allowances are only references; actual individual needs based upon starting nutritional status and special metabolic requirements, such as surgery, must be considered. Some individual variations may occur, and, therefore, any nutritional requirements above the DRI should be prescribed by a properly trained physician or nutritionist.

Caloric intake suggestions are also included in Chapter 2. These are based upon the caloric requirements to maintain a normal body weight in a person free of disease. Caloric requirements may increase with disease or surgery, and they may decrease with a more sedentary lifestyle. Therefore, caloric recommendations will depend upon the actual physical status of the individual.

Proper nutrition is an important factor in the maintenance of health and the prevention of disease. Compromised chewing capacity affects millions of Americans from all geographic regions and socioeconomic strata, and this group is more likely to suffer nutritional debility. The *I-Can't-Chew Cookbook* addresses both the nutritional and the gustatory requirements of the individual on a soft or liquid diet. I hope that it will stimulate the palates of those who otherwise are bored by their chewing restrictions, while it also improves or maintains the nutrition important for good health and recovery from surgery and disease.

— *Mark A. Piper, D.M.D., M.D.*
St. Petersburg, Florida

Preface

I developed the *I-Can't-Chew Cookbook* to provide recipes and hints helpful to those on a soft-food diet. It is my pleasure to share with you a new world of cooking and dining pleasure that is delightful for the entire family. I hope you enjoy the recipes as much as I have enjoyed compiling them.

Although I have never been a professional chef, I've always enjoyed developing nutritional meals that taste good. I am happy to have updated this cookbook since it was first published in 1985. I have improved the recipes and added new ones that the entire family can enjoy.

Good nutrition is very important for all of us, and the science that goes into determining what constitutes good nutrition is updated continually. Included in this edition of the *I-Can't-Chew Cookbook* is a chapter titled "The Science of Nutrition Today," by Linda Yoakam, a registered dietician. In it, she discusses the most recent nutritional guidelines that have been established for healthy adults. Her comments are supplemented by the chapters "More Nutritional Information" and "Tips for Getting the Most Out of Meals" (the latter was authored by Debra Mestas, R.D.).

Individuals on a restricted diet have a greater challenge than the rest of us to eat the variety of foods that most nutritionists agree is the first guideline for a balanced diet. That is where the *I-Can't-Chew Cookbook* can help. The recipes I have developed use foods from all the food groups. I haven't skipped vegetables and fruits, two types of food often problematic for those on a soft-food diet. For those on a restricted-sodium diet, I have eliminated salt where it does not dramatically enhance the flavor. When a recipe calls for salt, you may wish to omit the salt if your diet requires restricted sodium intake. Also, because dentists are adamant about the dangers of sugar to our teeth, and because some people need to cut sugar from their diet, we have used the sugar substitute Equal in many of our recipes and provide substitution information as appropriate. I have also included a nutritional analysis with each recipe. This will help you determine how the recipe contributes to overall nutrition. The nutritional analyses were computed using Nutritionist Pro software.

Perhaps you have your own favorite recipe or helpful hint for those on a soft-food diet. I invite you to share those with me. As I learn of new ideas and recipes, I may include them in future editions of the book. Please e-mail me with your hints and recipes. My e-mail address is randyw94@mymtnhome.com.

The recipes contained in this book will teach you new and creative ways to prepare food in accordance with a soft-food diet. However, they can also be enjoyed by the rest of the family. Delightful and nutritious recipes make eating enjoyable and good health attainable. I urge you to be creative with your daily diet, and I wish you the best of health and happy eating.

— *J. Randy Wilson*
May, 2003

Acknowledgments

I would like to give a special thanks to the following people who assisted me with this book. They gave their time, professional advice, and recipe suggestions.

Mark A. Piper, D.M.D., M.D., P.A.

Peter E. Dawson, D.D.S.

Jennifer Anderson, M.S., R.D.

James D. Cummins, D.D.S.

Ken Wiencek, D.D.S.

Bonnie Sherman, Home Economist

Debra Mestas, R.D.

Maggie Klink

Phyllis Hackett, R.N.

John Powers

Sue Spitler

Pat Molden

Linda Yoakam, M.S., R.D., L.D.

A Note Regarding Sugar and Equal

Dentists are adamant about the dangers of sugar to our teeth, so we have used Equal in many of our recipes. Since some people are adverse to using Equal because of other health reasons, recipes in which Equal can be used instead of sugar also inform the reader of how many Equal packets should be substituted for the sugar. Please note, though, that Equal is inappropriate for substitution for sugar in some recipes, as sugar provides qualities other than sweetening that Equal cannot provide, and such a substitution may change the texture or consistency of the recipe significantly.

Important Note

The material in this book is intended to provide recipes suitable for individuals on a soft-food diet. Every effort has been made to provide accurate and dependable information. The contents of this book have been compiled through professional research and in consultation with medical professionals. However, health-care professionals have differing opinions, and advances in medical and scientific research are made very quickly, so some of the information may become outdated.

Therefore, the publisher, authors, editors, and the professionals quoted in the book cannot be held responsible for any error, omission, or dated material. The authors and publisher assume no responsibility for any outcome of applying the information in this book in a program of self-care or under the care of a licensed practitioner. If you have questions concerning your nutrition or diet, or about the application of the information described in this book, consult a qualified health-care professional.

Chapter 1

◇ ◇ ◇

The Science of Nutrition Today

by Linda Yoakam, M.S., R.D., L.D.

Nutrition is an ever-growing science of how the body uses food. Experts in nutrition are continually learning more about the foods we eat. Not only how foods serve to maintain basic health, but also how these same foods can enhance health. Even for those restricted to a soft-foods diet it's possible—and equally necessary— to follow a health-promoting diet. Although it may require careful planning to do so, a soft-foods diet can include adequate amounts of all the vital nutrients and can adhere to generally accepted guidelines for healthful eating.

Experts in the science of nutrition have grouped nutrients into six classes. The three classes of nutrients that provide energy (calories) are the most abundant, were the first to be identified, and are the most well known of the nutrients; they are carbohydrates, proteins, and fats. In the twentieth century, particularly from the 1940s to 1960s, another class of nutrients was discovered: the vitamins. Vitamins are organic compounds necessary for life. They do not provide calories and are used by the body only in small amounts. There are fifteen known vitamins. Ten of them are described in the next chapter, "More Nutritional Information." The other five are easily obtained in a normal diet; deficiencies in them are rare or unknown. During the 1900s, research also occurred into the importance and roles of various minerals. There are thirteen essential minerals. The six major minerals in terms of amounts needed are described in the next chapter. And finally, but most importantly, there is the nutrient water. All six of these classes of nutrients are required to sustain and nurture life.

Basic Nutritional Guidelines

As the science of nutrition expanded to identify these essential nutrients, research continued in the area of how much of each nutrient is needed. Guidelines were first written for minimum intakes to prevent deficiency diseases. But intakes recommended for the prevention of disease were not thought to be enough to meet all of the body's needs, so in 1943, the RDAs (Recommended Dietary Allowances, written by the Food and Nutrition Board of the National Research Council) were established to maintain the health of a population group. The RDAs continued to be reviewed and rewritten as new research was made available; they were last rewritten and released in 1989. Now, for the twenty-first century, the guidelines come from the National Academy of Sciences' Institute of Medicine and are called the *Dietary Reference Intakes (DRIs)*. The DRIs are designed to meet the needs of individuals who are healthy and free of specific diseases or conditions that may alter their daily nutritional requirements. There are DRIs for all classes of nutrients, except water; different amounts are given for different age and sex categories. DRIs for healthy adult women and men are included in the next chapter.

All of this is a lot to remember for any individual deciding what to eat at any particular meal. No single food provides all the needed nutrients. The variety of nutrients required by the body needs to come from a variety of foods. To help in the selection of a healthy variety of foods, several guides have been developed. The USDA Food Guide Pyramid is the current recommended guideline for Americans.

The pyramid divides foods into six groups, based on the types of nutrients they contain. These groups are listed below (recommended serving sizes of the various foods are included in parentheses):

Bread group—Includes breads (1 slice), ready-to-eat cereals (1 ounce), cooked cereals ($\frac{1}{2}$ cup), cooked rice or pasta ($\frac{1}{2}$ cup). These foods are rich in B vitamins, iron, fiber, and complex carbohydrates. Six to eleven servings per day are recommended. These foods form the base, or foundation, of the pyramid, because they should form the base, or foundation, of a healthy daily diet.

A Guide to Daily Food Choices

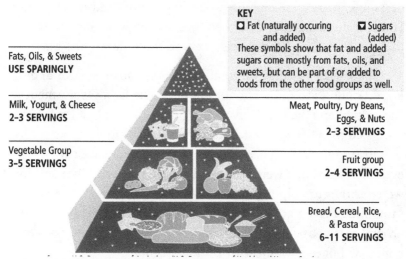

KEY
◻ Fat (naturally occuring   ▽ Sugars
and added)   (added)
These symbols show that fat and added sugars come mostly from fats, oils, and sweets, but can be part of or added to foods from the other food groups as well.

Fats, Oils, & Sweets
USE SPARINGLY

Milk, Yogurt, & Cheese
2-3 SERVINGS

Meat, Poultry, Dry Beans,
Eggs, & Nuts
2-3 SERVINGS

Vegetable Group
3-5 SERVINGS

Fruit group
2-4 SERVINGS

Bread, Cereal, Rice,
& Pasta Group
6-11 SERVINGS

(Source: U.S. Department of Agriculture/U.S.Department of Health and Human Services)

Vegetable group—Includes all cooked or chopped raw vegetables (½ cup), and raw leafy vegetables (1 cup). Vegetables are good sources of many vitamins and minerals, particularly vitamin A, vitamin C, folate, and dietary fiber. Three to five servings daily are recommended.

Fruit group—Includes all fresh (1 piece), frozen or canned fruits (½ cup), and fruit juices (½ cup). Like vegetables, fruits are good sources of a variety of vitamins and minerals, as well as fiber. Two to four servings per day are recommended. Fruits, with vegetables, form the second layer of a good diet.

Milk, yogurt, and cheese group—Includes milk or yogurt (8 fluid ounces), and hard or soft cheeses (1 or 1½ ounces). Foods in this group provide protein, calcium, riboflavin, vitamin D, and other minerals. Two to three servings daily are recommended.

Meat, poultry, fish, dry beans, eggs, and nuts group—Two to three servings daily are recommended of these protein-rich foods that also provide zinc, iron, and other nutrients. One serving is two to three ounces, much less than what is consumed in the typical American diet. That is why this group makes up a much smaller portion of the pyramid.

Fats, oils, and sweets group—This group includes cooking oils, salad dressings, margarine or butter, desserts, candy, and other sweets. Foods from this group should be used sparingly as they contribute to illnesses such as heart disease, cancer, tooth decay, and obesity.

The science of nutrition continues to expand. The DRIs and the Food Guide Pyramid were not enough. The U.S. Department of Agriculture and the U.S. Department of Health and Human Services produced the Dietary Guidelines for Americans to promote the use of nutrition to prevent diseases. The Dietary Guidelines are revised every five years, and were last issued in 2000. The current guidelines were written to help people find ways to enjoy food while at the same time taking action to promote good health. They are built around three basic messages, with several specific suggestions contained within each of those three fundamentals:

A—Aim for fitness:

- Aim for a healthy weight.
- Be physically active each day.

B—Build a healthy base:

- Let the pyramid guide your food choices.
- Choose a variety of grains daily, especially whole grains.
- Keep food safe to eat.

C—Choose sensibly:

- Choose a diet that is low in saturated fat and cholesterol and moderate in total fat.
- Choose beverages and foods to moderate your intake of sugars.
- Choose and prepare foods with less salt.
- If you drink alcoholic beverages, do so in moderation.

Today, research is also occurring in the areas of phytonutrients and probiotics. The term *phytonutrients* refers to organic compounds in foods (just like vitamins) that are *not* essential (unlike vitamins, which *are* essential), but are thought to be good for health. Examples of phytonutrients include isoflavones (estrogen-like compounds contained in soy foods) and carotenoids (which give color to fruits and vegetables, and may protect against heart disease, some cancers, and macular degeneration). Much further research in this area needs to be undertaken, but studies so far are promising. For now, consumption of phytonutrient-rich foods such as fruits, vegetables, grains, and tea would be prudent.

The term *probiotics* refers to the beneficial or "good" bacteria naturally occurring in foods. A possibility exists that these may help prevent or treat such bacterial illnesses as vaginal yeast infections and diarrhea. Initial studies have shown mixed results, but nutrition is an evolving science.

Chewing Difficulties May Mean Different Nutritional Needs

The basic health principles established in the DRIs, the Food Guide Pyramid, the U.S. Dietary Guidelines, and the new areas of phytonutrients and probiotics are applicable regardless of one's ability to chew food. However, all these guidelines were written to apply to essentially healthy individuals and to prevent the sorts of "lifestyle-related" illnesses that are the most common causes of death and chronic poor health in the United States—conditions such as obesity, heart disease, stroke, diabetes, and certain types of cancer. Chewing or swallowing difficulties can develop with oral surgery, worn or poor-fitting dentures, cancers and their therapies, temporomandibular joint syndrome (TMJS), or as a result of stroke, multiple sclerosis, Parkinson's disease, Alzheimer's disease, and a host of other illnesses. An individual suffering from one of these conditions may have nutritional needs that differ somewhat from the goals of the guidelines outlined above. A cancer patient undergoing chemotherapy, for example, may need to focus more than the average person on boosting calories and protein intake. General suggestions for how to modify cooking and eating habits to accommodate difficulties chewing and swallowing—including pointers for boosting calories, protein, and fiber—are provided in Chapter 3, "Tips for Getting the Most Out of Meals." If you are restricted in your ability to chew, consult with your doctor or a dietician or nutritionist about your particular dietary needs. Do you need to concentrate on eating as much food as you can? Or, like most Americans, do you need to be careful to avoid exceeding a healthy caloric intake? A diet that does not require chewing can be just as healthy as one that does require chewing. Whatever your specific nutritional needs, this book aims to help you achieve a healthy diet.

Chapter 2

More Nutritional Information

Major Nutrients: Their Functions, Food Sources, and Dietary Reference Intakes (DRIs)

Nutrient	Function in the Body	Food Sources	DRI Women	DRI Men
Protein	Basic building block of all tissues. Builds and repairs all body tissues. Supplies energy. Helps form antibodies, which fight infection.	Meat, fish, poultry, eggs, milk, cheese, dried peas and beans, soybeans and soy products, nuts, cereals, breads.	10–35% of daily caloric intake*	10–35% of daily caloric intake*
Carbohydrate	Supplies energy for heat and mechanical work.	Sugars, fruits, vegetables, cereals, breads, rice, pasta.	45–65% of daily caloric intake*	45–65% of daily caloric intake*
Fat	Supplies energy to do physical work. Major storage form of excess energy in the body. Aids in absorption of vitamins A, D, E, and K, and calcium.	Margarine, vegetable oils, butter, salad dressings, fatty meats, whole-milk products, egg yolks, nuts, cheese, bacon, shortening, lard.	20–35% of daily caloric intake*	20–35% of daily caloric intake*

Nutrient	Function in the Body	Food Sources	DRI Women	DRI Men
Vitamin A	Promotes normal vision in dim light. Promotes healthy skin and tissue lining. Helps maintain resistance to infection.	Liver, eggs, dark green and yellow vegetables, butter, margarine, peaches, cantaloupe, apricots, whole milk products, low-fat milk with vitamin A added, fish liver oils.	700 RE	900 RE
Thiamin or vitamin B-1	Promotes normal digestion, growth, and appetite. Helps keep the nervous system healthy. Helps change food into energy.	Pork; liver; heart; kidney; dried peas and beans; nuts; wheat germ; whole-grain, restored, enriched, and fortified cereals and breads.	1.1 mg	1.2 mg
Riboflavin or vitamin B-2	Necessary for the release of energy from food. Helps keep eyes, mouth, and skin healthy. Promotes vitality and growth.	Beef, pork, lamb, liver, milk and milk products, yogurt, eggs, green leafy vegetables, cheese, peanuts, enriched and fortified cereals and breads.	1.1 mg	1.3 mg
Niacin	Helps keep skin, mouth, and nervous system healthy. Helps convert food into energy. Aids in digestion.	Lean meat; fish; poultry; liver; kidney; peanuts; peanut butter; mushrooms; dried peas and beans; whole-grain, restored, enriched, and fortified cereals and breads.	14 mg	16 mg

Nutrient	Function in the Body	Food Sources	DRI Women	DRI Men
Vitamin B-6	Aids in digestion of protein.	Meat, fish, chicken, liver, egg yolks, peanuts, peanut butter, bananas, potatoes, corn, whole-grain and fortified cereals and breads.	1.5 mg	1.7 mg
Vitamin B-12	Necessary for proper functioning of all cells.	Meat, fish, liver, kidney, eggs, milk, cheese, fortified cereals.	2.4 µg	2.4 µg
Folic acid (folate)	Necessary for the formation of blood cells. Coenzyme in the metabolism of nucleic and amino acids. Prevents megaloblastic anemia.	Liver, dried beans, peanuts, walnuts, filberts, dark green vegetables, fortified cereals.	400 µg	400 µg
Vitamin C or ascorbic acid	Important for healthy tissues, gums, blood vessels, bones, and teeth. Helps promote healing, stamina, and energy.	Citrus fruits and juices, strawberries, cantaloupe, broccoli, cabbage, tomatoes, tomato juice, bell peppers, potatoes, leafy greens, watermelon, Brussels sprouts.	75 mg	90 mg
Vitamin D	Aids in absorption of calcium and phosphorus, which build and maintain bones and teeth.	Fish liver oils, fortified milk, liver, egg yolks, herring, mackerel, canned salmon, sardines, sunshine.	10 µg	10 µg
Vitamin E	Important for the stability of substances in the body tissues.	Liver, eggs, whole-grain cereals and breads, whole milk, margarine, salad oil, salad dressing, green leafy vegetables.	15 mg	15 mg

Nutrient	Function in the Body	Food Sources	DRI Women	DRI Men
Calcium	Needed to build bones and teeth. Helps nerves, muscles, and heart function properly. Helps blood clotting.	Milk and milk products, canned salmon with bones, sardines, green leafy vegetables.	1,200 mg	1,200 mg
Iron	Helps build red blood cells.	Meat; liver; egg yolks; tuna; oysters; green leafy vegetables; dried fruits; whole-grain, restored, enriched, and fortified cereals and breads.	18 mg	8 mg
Phosphorus	Needed to build bones and teeth.	Meat, fish, poultry, eggs, dried beans, peanuts, whole-grain cereals and breads, milk and milk products.	700 mg	700 mg
Magnesium	Needed for proper functioning of body cells.	Dried beans, nuts, dark green vegetables, whole-grain cereals and breads.	320 mg	420 mg
Iodine	Needed to help regulate many body functions.	Iodized salt, seafood.	150 µg	150 µg
Zinc	Needed for growth and development, and for synthesis of collagen and DNA. Important for wound healing and immune function.	Seafood, turkey, meat, liver, egg yolk, whole-grain products, molasses, seeds, wheat germ, brewer's yeast, milk.	8 mg	11 mg

mg = milligrams   µg = micrograms   RE = retinol equivalent

*To calculate daily recommended grams of protein, carbs, or fat based on this percentage, take the total calories per day times the percent given divided by 4 (for protein), 4 (for carbs), or 9 (for fat). In other words, if you are supposed in ingest 2000 calories per day and want to figure out how many grams of carbohydrates you should consume, do the following: 2000 X 50% = 1000 / 4 = 250 gm.

Body Mass Index (BMI)

The body mass index (BMI) is a measurement of weight as it compares to height. Instead of height/weight tables, BMI is the measurement now used by most nutritionists, medical researchers, and government agencies to determine whether an individual's weight is appropriate for his or her height.

Use the following steps to calculate your BMI:

⬦ Divide your weight in pounds by your height in inches (e.g., 140 ÷ 65 = 2.154)

⬦ Divide that number again by your height in inches (2.154 ÷ 65 = 0.0331)

⬦ Multiply that number by 703 (0.0331 x 703 = 23.27)

⬦ Locate your results below:

> Below 18.5—underweight
>
> 18.5 to 24.9—healthy weight
>
> 25 to 29.9—overweight
>
> 30 to 39.9—obese
>
> 40+—severely obese

(Children and pregnant women have different BMI guidelines.)

The drawback with BMI is that it fails to take into account one's body composition—that is, the ratio of muscle to fat. For that reason, a professional athlete may register a BMI above 25, not because he or she needs to lose weight but rather because his or her body composition has an unusually high percentage of muscle. Nevertheless, in terms of health, BMI is a useful guide for most adults.

Table of Body Mass Indexes

BMI (kg/m2)	19	20	21	22	23	24	25	26	27	28	29	30	35	40
Height (in.)	Body Weight (lbs.)													
58	91	96	100	105	110	115	119	124	129	134	138	143	167	191
59	94	99	104	109	114	119	124	128	133	138	143	148	173	198
60	97	102	107	112	118	123	128	133	138	143	148	153	179	204
61	100	106	111	116	122	127	132	137	143	148	153	158	185	211
62	104	109	115	120	126	131	136	142	147	153	158	164	191	218
63	107	113	118	124	130	135	141	146	152	158	163	169	197	225
64	110	116	122	128	134	140	145	151	157	163	169	174	204	232
65	114	120	126	132	138	144	150	156	162	168	174	180	210	240
66	118	124	130	136	142	148	155	161	167	173	179	186	216	247
67	121	127	134	140	146	153	159	166	172	178	185	191	223	255
68	125	131	138	144	151	158	164	171	177	184	190	197	230	262
69	128	135	142	149	155	162	169	176	182	189	196	203	236	270
70	132	139	146	153	160	167	174	181	188	195	202	207	243	278
71	136	143	150	157	165	172	179	186	193	200	208	215	250	286
72	140	147	154	162	169	177	184	191	199	206	213	221	258	294
73	144	151	159	166	174	182	189	197	204	212	219	227	265	302
74	148	155	163	171	179	186	194	202	210	218	225	233	272	311
75	152	160	168	176	184	192	200	208	216	224	232	240	279	319
76	156	164	172	180	189	197	205	213	221	230	238	246	287	328

(Source: Consumer.gov, a resource for consumer information sponsored by the U.S. federal government: www.consumer.gov/weightloss/bmi.htm.)

Calorie Recommendations

Recommendations for calories were revised with the Fall 2002 publication of the DRIs. These are for people of normal weight; they are not designed for use with a weight-loss program. The caloric recommendations given below are based multiple factors, including age, sex, weight, and, new to this edition, activity level. There are four levels of physical activity in the new guidelines: Sedentary, or about the same as resting; Low Activity, or only using about 10 percent more calories over resting; Active, or using slightly under 25 percent more calories than resting; and Very Active, or using almost 50 percent more calories than resting. Increasing one's activity or exercise level to meet the Active calorie level improves cardiovascular and overall health and allows for plenty of healthy food choices. The recommended calorie intakes for Active people are listed below:

Female

1–3 years	992 cal
4–8 years	1,642 cal
9–13 years	2,071 cal
14–18 years	2,368 cal
>19–years	2,403 cal (subtract 7 cal per day for each year above 19)

Male

1–3 years	1,046 cal
4–8 years	1,742 cal
9–13 years	2,279 cal
14–18 years	3,152 cal
>19–years	3,069 cal (subtract 10 cal/day for each year above 19)

Chapter 3

◇ ◇ ◇

Tips for
Getting the Most
Out of Meals

Dealing with Problems Swallowing and/or Chewing

by Debra Mestas, R.D.

When swallowing or chewing is made difficult because of dental or medical problems, it is easy to get into a habit of limiting food selections. An inadequate diet often occurs in these situations. To maintain adequate nutrition under such circumstances, consider the following recommendations:

◇ Cut or grind food into appropriate-size pieces, and put them into a cream sauce or mix them with other foods, as in a casserole

◇ Make rich soups of creamed or blended meats and vegetables, or of dried beans, peas, lentils, or soybeans

◇ Add eggs and cheese to increase protein

◇ Use mashed or puréed fruits and vegetables or their juices

◇ Cook hot cereals in milk instead of water

◇ Use gelatins, ice creams, puddings, custards, and milk shakes

To Boost Protein

◇ Add dry skim-milk powder to regular milk, sauces, gravies, and puddings. Add extra ice cream to shakes, and half-and-half or evaporated milk to instant cocoa, soups, or puddings

◇ Add grated cheese to casseroles, vegetables, sauces. Blended cottage cheese makes a great dip

◇ Add finely chopped eggs to sauces, casseroles, and meat salads. Prepare beverages and desserts that use eggs, such as eggnogs or angel food cake

◇ Add chopped or puréed meats to soups and casseroles

To Boost Calories

◇ Melt margarine or butter onto hot toast, cereals, vegetables, rice, or eggs

◇ Use sour cream on potatoes, meats, or fruits

◇ Use cream cheese on bread and fruit

◇ Use mayonnaise instead of salad dressings

◇ Put peanut butter on apples, bananas, celery, carrots, and breads

◇ Top puddings, pies, hot chocolate, gelatin, and fruit with whipped cream

◇ Use honey, candies, and jelly, but only as a supplement to nutritious foods

To Boost Fiber

◇ Use whole-grain breads and cereals

◇ Use unpeeled apples and potatoes

◇ Eat oranges and grapefruit and their unstrained juices

◇ Add sunflower, sesame, poppy, or pumpkin seeds to salads, breads, and other foods

- Make soups with dried beans, peas, lentils, or soybeans

- Add dates, raisins, figs, or dried apricots to hot cereals, cakes, and muffins

- Make carrot or cabbage slaw with pineapple and raisins

- Add broccoli, cauliflower, and corn to soups and casseroles

- Top sandwiches and salads with alfalfa or bean sprouts

- Eat more sliced tomatoes, and use more tomatoes in sauces and soups

- Snack on popcorn

- Add fresh parsley to salads

Enhancing the Dining Experience

Besides following specially adapted recipes, there are ways to increase mealtime enjoyment despite the restrictions imposed by a soft-food diet. The following are some pointers to consider:

Pay attention to atmosphere: A table set attractively with candles, flowers, or a decorative centerpiece can make any meal more enjoyable. So can dining with friends, playing background music at mealtime, and varying the place in your house where you eat.

Make up your own recipes: Try ice cream or sherbet mixed with ginger ale or your favorite carbonated beverage. Create your own version of a milk shake, frozen yogurt, or eggnog.

Eat a number of small meals during the day.

Vary the color of foods served: Arrange the food attractively on the plate. Add garnishes, such as an orange wedge, a slice of tomato, a sprig of parsley, or a sprinkling of chopped cilantro.

Purée foods in a blender or food processor: If you like soup, for example, heat it and then blend it. Food tastes better if it is cooked before it is blended, and it is also easier to blend warm food. Beware, however, of the fact that hot food expands suddenly when blended. To avoid a mini-explosion when you turn on the blender, blend food that's warm rather than hot, and blend only small amounts at a time. Cut meat into small pieces and add gravy prior to blending.

Serve soft foods: Try mashed potatoes, yogurt, scrambled eggs, poached eggs, egg custards, milk shakes, puddings, gelatins, creamy cereals, and ice cream.

Try tilting your head back or moving it forward to make swallowing easier.

Rinse your mouth regularly: Doing so will remove debris, stimulate your gums, lubricate your mouth, and put a fresh taste in your mouth.

Don't ignore your food cravings: If you're hankering after a favorite food that cannot be puréed, satisfy your desire by simply placing a small piece of the food in your mouth. That way, you still get to savor the flavor.

Serve baby food spiced with grown-up seasonings.

Adapting Foods for a Soft-Food Diet

Explore all types of beverages.

Bread and cereal products: Serve blended or strained and cooked cereals such as cream of wheat, farina, hominy grits, and oatmeal. Try macaroni, spaghetti, or noodles chopped into tiny pieces, as well as thoroughly cooked rice. Make sure enough liquid is added for a smooth consistency. Bran can be added to many foods to increase fiber.

Meat, poultry, fish, eggs, and cheese: Try blended or strained beef, lamb, pork, veal, fowl, and liver. Try eggs prepared any way but fried or hard boiled. Serve small-curd cottage cheese, cream cheese, or grated natural cheeses such as cheddar and swiss. Also, use prepared "toddler" baby foods.

Milk and milk products: All milk and milk products, such as ice cream, custards, and yogurt, are appropriate for a soft-food diet. To avoid constipation from overindulgence in dairy products, supplement the diet with bran.

Fruits: Enjoy all fruit juices and nectars; fresh canned or cooked fruit, such as peaches, pears, apples, apricots, bananas and cherries; and prepared "toddler" baby foods. Some fruits should be cooked before blending. Others, such as berries, work well when puréed with ice and other ingredients for smoothies. Very ripe fruits will blend best.

Vegetables: Most vegetables, if well cooked, can be served whole, and each bite can be mashed with a fork before eating it. This is much more appetizing than serving premashed vegetables. Try vegetable juices such as V-8, carrot, celery, and tomato. Consider investing in a juicer so you can make your own juice from fresh veggies. Also prepare cooked, mild-flavored puréed vegetables, such as asparagus, beans (green and wax), beets, carrots, peas, spinach, winter squash, and tomato purée. Mashed potatoes (white or sweet) work well, as do prepared "toddler" baby foods.

Soups: All meat broths are appropriate, as are all cream soups served with mashed potatoes, puréed vegetables, or strained meat.

Sweets and desserts: Try smooth-textured desserts such as custards, gelatin, ice cream, puddings, or sherbet. Enjoy chocolate milk, jellies, and syrups (such as chocolate, butterscotch, caramel, and marshmallow).

Fats: Enjoy butter, cream, margarine, and vegetable oils (but use sparingly!).

Condiments, spices, and sauces: Spice up your meals with variations on seasonings and condiments, including flavored catsups, mustards, marinades, spice rubs, fancy vinegars, pepper sauces, sesame oil, etc.

Commercial products: If you need a boost in calories and nutrients, try some of the supplemental meals on the market, for example, Instant Breakfast, Boost, Ensure, Glucerna (for diabetics), Meritene (powder or liquid), or Sustacal (powder or liquid), as well as prepared "toddler" baby foods.

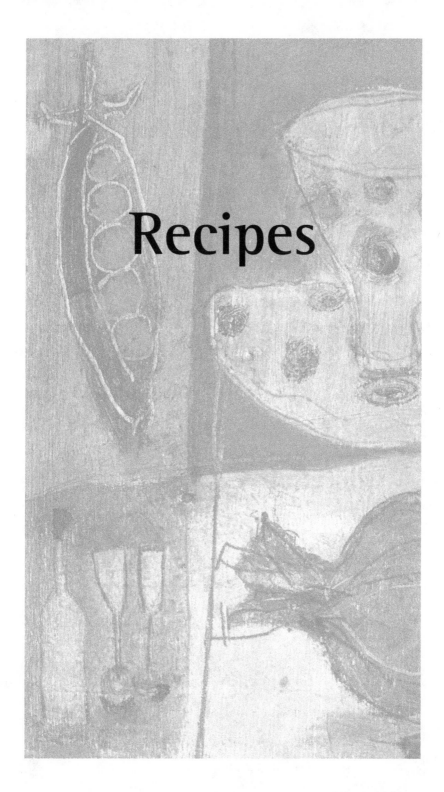

Recipes

Beverages

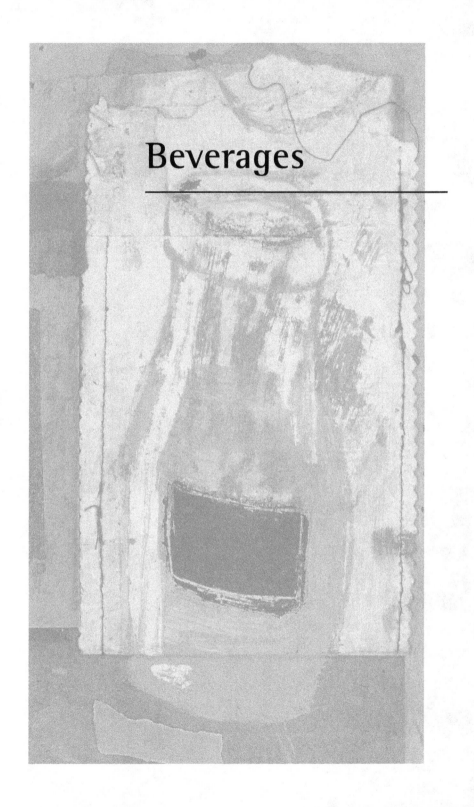

Limeade

PER SERVING: 169.8 CALORIES — 0.5 g PROTEIN — 46.5 g CARBOHYDRATE — 0.5 g FIBER — 0 g TOTAL FAT — 0 g SATURATED FAT — 0 mg CHOLESTEROL — 76.2 mg SODIUM

½ cup fresh lime juice
3–4 tablespoons sugar*
1½ cups club soda
Ice cubes

Combine lime juice and sugar in large glass, stirring until sugar is dissolved. Stir in club soda; add ice.

Makes 1 serving.

*Can substitute with 4 packets of Equal

Nutritional Analysis per Serving

Vitamin A	2.4 RE	Vitamin D	0.0 µg
Thiamin (B-1)	0.0 mg	Vitamin E	0.1 mg
Riboflavin (B-2)	0.0 mg	Calcium	26.7 mg
Niacin	0.1 mg	Iron	0.1 mg
Vitamin B-6	0.1 mg	Phosphorus	8.0 mg
Vitamin B-12	0.0 µg	Magnesium	10.9 mg
Folate (total)	15.9 µg	Zinc	0.4 mg
Vitamin C	56.1 mg	Potassium	159.1 mg

Old-Fashioned Lemonade

PER SERVING: 77.1 CALORIES — 0.2 g PROTEIN — 21.2 g CARBOHYDRATE — 0.2 g FIBER —
0 g TOTAL FAT — 0 g SATURATED FAT — 0 mg CHOLESTEROL — 0.8 mg SODIUM

1 cup fresh lemon juice

$^1/_3$–$^1/_2$ cup sugar*

4 cups cold water

1 lemon, sliced

Ice cubes

Combine the lemon juice and sugar in pitcher and stir until sugar dissolves. Stir in water and lemon slices; serve over ice.

Makes 4 servings.

*Can substitute with 4 packets of Equal

Nutritional Analysis per Serving

Vitamin A	1.2 RE	Vitamin D	0.0 µg
Thiamin (B-1)	0.0 mg	Vitamin E	0.1 mg
Riboflavin (B-2)	0.0 mg	Calcium	4.4 mg
Niacin	0.1 mg	Iron	0.0 mg
Vitamin B-6	0.0 mg	Phosphorus	4.0 mg
Vitamin B-12	0.0 µg	Magnesium	3.7 mg
Folate (total)	7.9 µg	Zinc	0.0 mg
Vitamin C	28.1 mg	Potassium	76.0 mg

Minted Pineapple Cooler

PER SERVING: 153.0 CALORIES — 0.5 g PROTEIN — 39.3 g CARBOHYDRATE — 1.6 g FIBER —
0.5 g TOTAL FAT — 0.0 g SATURATED FAT — 0 mg CHOLESTEROL — 2.0 mg SODIUM

1 medium fresh pineapple, peeled, cored, finely chopped (about 3 cups)

2 cups water

$1/2$ cup sugar*

$1/4$ cup fresh mint leaves

2 tablespoons lime juice

Place pineapple in medium sauce pan. Add water and sugar. Heat to boiling; reduce heat and simmer, covered, 15 minutes. Stir in mint. Let stand, covered, about 1 hour or until cool. Strain; discard mint leaves and reserve pineapple for another use. Stir lime juice into pineapple liquid. Refrigerate until chilled. Serve over ice cubes. Add sugar and stir until dissolved just before serving.

Makes 4 servings.

TIP: Reserved pineapple makes a delicious topping for ice cream or pound cake.

*Can substitute with 15 packets of Equal

Nutritional Analysis per Serving

Vitamin A	9.2 RE	Vitamin D	0.0 µg
Thiamin (B-1)	0.1 mg	Vitamin E	0.1 mg
Riboflavin (B-2)	0.1 mg	Calcium	13.0 mg
Niacin	0.5 mg	Iron	0.5 mg
Vitamin B-6	0.1 mg	Phosphorus	10.3 mg
Vitamin B-12	0.0 µg	Magnesium	18.0 mg
Folate (total)	15.2 µg	Zinc	0.1 mg
Vitamin C	20.7 mg	Potassium	149.3 mg

Cranberry Orange Tea

PER SERVING: 61.5 CALORIES — 0 g PROTEIN — 15.5 g CARBOHYDRATE — 0.1 g FIBER —
0.1 g TOTAL FAT — 0 g SATURATED FAT — 0 mg CHOLESTEROL — 3.5 mg SODIUM

3$\frac{1}{2}$ cups water
2$\frac{1}{2}$ cups cranberry juice cocktail
8 orange flavor herb tea bags

Heat water and cranberry juice to boiling in large saucepan. Remove from heat. Add tea bags; let stand, covered, 5 minutes. Remove tea bags.

Makes 6 servings.

Nutritional Analysis per Serving

Vitamin A	0.0 RE	Vitamin D	0.0 µg
Thiamin (B-1)	0.0 mg	Vitamin E	0.0 mg
Riboflavin (B-2)	0.0 mg	Calcium	5.9 mg
Niacin	0.0 mg	Iron	0.3 mg
Vitamin B-6	0.0 mg	Phosphorus	2.1 mg
Vitamin B-12	0.0 µg	Magnesium	3.5 mg
Folate (total)	1.4 µg	Zinc	0.1 mg
Vitamin C	37.3 mg	Potassium	31.4 mg

Fresh Orange Milk Shake

PER SERVING: 203.8 CALORIES — 3.0 g PROTEIN — 34.2 g CARBOHYDRATE — 0.5 g FIBER —
6.5 g TOTAL FAT — 3.7 g SATURATED FAT — 22.6 mg CHOLESTEROL — 23.3 mg SODIUM

2 cups fresh orange juice

$1/2$ cup vanilla ice cream

$1/2$ teaspoon vanilla

Process all ingredients in blender or food processor until smooth.
Makes 2 servings.

Nutritional Analysis per Serving

Vitamin A	117.7 RE	Vitamin D	0.0 µg
Thiamin (B-1)	0.2 mg	Vitamin E	0.2 mg
Riboflavin (B-2)	0.1 mg	Calcium	70.7 mg
Niacin	1.0 mg	Iron	0.5 mg
Vitamin B-6	0.1 mg	Phosphorus	77.4 mg
Vitamin B-12	0.1 µg	Magnesium	31.5 mg
Folate (total)	76.3 µg	Zinc	0.3 mg
Vitamin C	124.3 mg	Potassium	556.4 mg

Sparkling Fruit Punch

PER SERVING: 74.6 CALORIES — 0.5 g PROTEIN — 18.3 g CARBOHYDRATE — 0.8 g FIBER —
0.2 g TOTAL FAT — 0 g SATURATED FAT — 0 mg CHOLESTEROL — 2.1 mg SODIUM

1½ cups boiling water
8 orange flavor herb tea bags
1 can (46-ounce) pineapple juice, chilled
2 cups strawberries, puréed
2 cups chilled seltzer water

Pour boiling water over tea bags in medium teapot or saucepan; cover and let stand 5 minutes. Remove tea bags; allow tea to cool. Refrigerate until cold. Combine tea, pineapple juice, and strawberries in punch bowl; stir in seltzer water.

Makes 12 servings.

Nutritional Analysis per Serving

Vitamin A	0.7 RE	Vitamin D	0.0 µg
Thiamin (B-1)	0.1 mg	Vitamin E	0.1 mg
Riboflavin (B-2)	0.0 mg	Calcium	29.8 mg
Niacin	0.4 mg	Iron	0.4 mg
Vitamin B-6	0.1 mg	Phosphorus	14.1 mg
Vitamin B-12	0.0 µg	Magnesium	18.3 mg
Folate (total)	32.2 µg	Zinc	0.2 mg
Vitamin C	26.4 mg	Potassium	203.0 mg

Mango Frappé

PER SERVING: 137.7 CALORIES — 2.7 g PROTEIN — 30.7 g CARBOHYDRATE — 2.3 g FIBER —
1.5 g TOTAL FAT — 0.8 g SATURATED FAT — 4.9 mg CHOLESTEROL — 33.2 mg SODIUM

1 1/2 cups chopped mangoes
1/2 cup 2% reduced-fat milk
1 tablespoon sugar*
1 tablespoon lime juice
1/4 teaspoon vanilla
6 ice cubes

Process mangoes, milk, sugar, lime juice, and vanilla in blender
or food processor until smooth. Add ice cubes and process until
thick and slushy.

Makes 2 servings.

TIP: Bananas, peaches, or other fresh fruit may be substituted
for the mangoes. Frozen fruit may also be used.

*Can substitute 3 packets of Equal

Nutritional Analysis per Serving (with Mango)

Vitamin A	516.2 RE	Vitamin D	0.6 µg
Thiamin (B-1)	0.1 mg	Vitamin E	1.4 mg
Riboflavin (B-2)	0.2 mg	Calcium	87.6 mg
Niacin	0.8 mg	Iron	0.2 mg
Vitamin B-6	0.2 mg	Phosphorus	72.3 mg
Vitamin B-12	0.2 µg	Magnesium	20.2 mg
Folate (total)	21.0 µg	Zinc	0.3 mg
Vitamin C	37.1 mg	Potassium	296.3 mg

Tofu Smoothie

PER SERVING: 168.9 CALORIES — 6.8 g PROTEIN — 33.3 g CARBOHYDRATE — 1.4 g FIBER —
1.3 g TOTAL FAT — 0.1 g SATURATED FAT — 4.0 mg CHOLESTEROL — 59.2 mg SODIUM

1/2 cup silken tofu
1 small banana or other fruit
1 carton (6 ounces) fat-free sugar-free fruit yogurt (any flavor)
1 teaspoon lemon juice
1 tablespoon honey
1/4–1/2 cup fat-free milk
4–6 ice cubes
Ground cinnamon, as garnish

Process tofu, banana, yogurt, lemon juice, and honey in food processor or blender until smooth, adding enough milk to bring to desired consistency. Add ice cubes; process until cubes are finely crushed. Sprinkle with cinnamon.

Makes 2 servings.

Nutritional Analysis per Serving

Vitamin A	23.5 RE	Vitamin D	0.3 µg
Thiamin (B-1)	0.1 mg	Vitamin E	1.1 mg
Riboflavin (B-2)	0.2 mg	Calcium	138.5 mg
Niacin	3.9 mg	Iron	0.6 mg
Vitamin B-6	0.4 mg	Phosphorus	97.8 mg
Vitamin B-12	0.4 µg	Magnesium	38.2 mg
Folate (total)	13.3 µg	Zinc	0.8 mg
Vitamin C	6.9 mg	Potassium	415.8 mg

Butterscotch Milk Shake

PER SERVING: 370.1 CALORIES — 11.9 g PROTEIN — 53.7 g CARBOHYDRATE — 0 g FIBER —
12.4 g TOTAL FAT — 7.7 g SATURATED FAT — 50.0 mg CHOLESTEROL — 279.0 mg SODIUM

1 cup fat-free milk
1/2 cup vanilla ice cream
1/2 teaspoon vanilla
2 tablespoons butterscotch syrup

Process all ingredients in blender or food processor until smooth.
Makes 1 serving.
TIP: Use any favorite flavor of ice cream syrup.

Nutritional Analysis per Serving

Vitamin A	285.6 RE	Vitamin D	2.5 µg
Thiamin (B-1)	0.1 mg	Vitamin E	0.1 mg
Riboflavin (B-2)	0.5 mg	Calcium	408.2 mg
Niacin	0.3 mg	Iron	0.1 mg
Vitamin B-6	0.1 mg	Phosphorus	317.9 mg
Vitamin B-12	1.2 µg	Magnesium	35.3 mg
Folate (total)	16.0 µg	Zinc	1.3 mg
Vitamin C	3.0 mg	Potassium	527.5 mg

Strawberry Milk Shake

PER SERVING: 242.8 CALORIES — 7.2 g PROTEIN — 27.6 g CARBOHYDRATE — 1.7 g FIBER —
12.5 g TOTAL FAT — 7.5 g SATURATED FAT — 47.6 mg CHOLESTEROL — 105.9 mg SODIUM

½ cup strawberries
½ cup vanilla ice cream
½ cup fat-free milk

Process all ingredients in blender or food processor until smooth.
Makes 1 serving.

Nutritional Analysis per Serving

Vitamin A	213.0 RE	Vitamin D	1.2 µg
Thiamin (B-1)	0.1 mg	Vitamin E	0.2 mg
Riboflavin (B-2)	0.3 mg	Calcium	247.3 mg
Niacin	0.3 mg	Iron	0.4 mg
Vitamin B-6	0.1 mg	Phosphorus	207.7 mg
Vitamin B-12	0.7 µg	Magnesium	28.8 mg
Folate (total)	22.8 µg	Zinc	0.9 mg
Vitamin C	42.6 mg	Potassium	440.5 mg

Berry Smoothie

PER SERVING: 198.9 CALORIES — 6.4 g PROTEIN — 38.5 g CARBOHYDRATE — 2.0 g FIBER —
2.6 g TOTAL FAT — 1.6 g SATURATED FAT — 10.2 mg CHOLESTEROL — 84.4 mg SODIUM

1 cup strawberries

1 package (10 ounces) frozen raspberries

1$^1/_2$ cups 2% reduced-fat milk

1 container (8 ounces) low-fat vanilla yogurt

$^1/_4$ cup honey

$^1/_2$ teaspoon vanilla extract

Ground nutmeg, as garnish

Process all ingredients, except nutmeg, in food processor or blender until smooth. Pour into glasses; sprinkle lightly with nutmeg. Makes 4 servings.

Nutritional Analysis per Serving

Vitamin A	60.6 RE	Vitamin D	0.9 µg
Thiamin (B-1)	0.1 mg	Vitamin E	0.1 mg
Riboflavin (B-2)	0.3 mg	Calcium	214.9 mg
Niacin	0.3 mg	Iron	0.5 mg
Vitamin B-6	0.1 mg	Phosphorus	171.2 mg
Vitamin B-12	0.6 µg	Magnesium	26.0 mg
Folate (total)	17.7 µg	Zinc	0.9 mg
Vitamin C	23.3 mg	Potassium	336.5 mg

Banana Milk Shake

PER SERVING: 260.4 CALORIES — 9.2 g PROTEIN — 39.2 g CARBOHYDRATE — 2.8 g FIBER —
8.7 g TOTAL FAT — 5.3 g SATURATED FAT — 34.2 mg CHOLESTEROL — 120.8 mg SODIUM

1 ripe banana, sliced
1 cup whole milk
1/4 teaspoon vanilla

Process all ingredients in blender or food processor until smooth.
Makes 1 serving.

Nutritional Analysis per Serving

Vitamin A	85.1 RE	Vitamin D	2.4 µg
Thiamin (B-1)	0.1 mg	Vitamin E	0.6 mg
Riboflavin (B-2)	0.5 mg	Calcium	297.6 mg
Niacin	0.8 mg	Iron	0.5 mg
Vitamin B-6	0.8 mg	Phosphorus	250.6 mg
Vitamin B-12	0.9 µg	Magnesium	66.1 mg
Folate (total)	34.6 µg	Zinc	1.1 mg
Vitamin C	12.9 mg	Potassium	839.7 mg

Lime-Strawberry Slush

PER SERVING: 131.1 CALORIES — 0.7 g PROTEIN — 34.6 g CARBOHYDRATE — 1.9 g FIBER —
0.3 g TOTAL FAT — 0 g SATURATED FAT — 0 mg CHOLESTEROL — 1.6 mg SODIUM

1/4 cup fresh lime juice
1/2 cup sliced strawberries
2–3 tablespoons sugar*
1 cup ice cubes

Process all ingredients in blender or food processor until slushy.
Makes 1 serving.

*Can substitute with 5 packets of Equal

Nutritional Analysis per Serving

Vitamin A	2.8 RE	Vitamin D	0.0 µg
Thiamin (B-1)	0.0 mg	Vitamin E	0.2 mg
Riboflavin (B-2)	0.1 mg	Calcium	15.9 mg
Niacin	0.2 mg	Iron	0.3 mg
Vitamin B-6	0.1 mg	Phosphorus	18.5 mg
Vitamin B-12	0.0 µg	Magnesium	10.9 mg
Folate (total)	17.9 µg	Zinc	0.1 mg
Vitamin C	58.9 mg	Potassium	187.1 mg

Spicy Banana Shake

PER SERVING: 114.2 CALORIES — 0.9 g PROTEIN — 29.6 g CARBOHYDRATE — 2.1 g FIBER —
0.4 g TOTAL FAT — 0.2 g SATURATED FAT — 0 mg CHOLESTEROL — 2.2 mg SODIUM

1$\frac{1}{2}$ cups boiling water
6 spiced herb tea bags
3 ripe bananas
2 tablespoons honey
1$\frac{1}{2}$ cups ice cubes

Pour boiling water over tea bags in teapot or medium saucepan; let stand covered 5 minutes. Remove tea bags; allow tea to cool. Process tea, bananas, and honey in blender or food processor until smooth. Add ice cubes and process until slushy.

Makes 4 servings.

Nutritional Analysis per Serving

Vitamin A	7.1 RE	Vitamin D	0.0 µg
Thiamin (B-1)	0.0 mg	Vitamin E	0.2 mg
Riboflavin (B-2)	0.1 mg	Calcium	7.7 mg
Niacin	0.5 mg	Iron	0.4 mg
Vitamin B-6	0.5 mg	Phosphorus	18.1 mg
Vitamin B-12	0.0 µg	Magnesium	26.8 mg
Folate (total)	17.9 µg	Zinc	0.2 mg
Vitamin C	8.1 mg	Potassium	363.9 mg

Mocha Frost

PER SERVING: 378.3 CALORIES — 16.5 g PROTEIN — 57.4 g CARBOHYDRATE — 0 g FIBER —
7.9 g TOTAL FAT — 2.8 g SATURATED FAT — 24.9 mg CHOLESTEROL — 279.9 mg SODIUM

2 cups fat-free milk
$^1/_3$ cup flavored instant coffee
1 cup strong coffee, cooled
1 cup vanilla or chocolate reduced-fat ice cream

Place all ingredients into blender and blend until smooth.
Makes 2 servings.

Nutritional Analysis per Serving

Vitamin A	239.5 RE	Vitamin D	2.5 µg
Thiamin (B-1)	0.1 mg	Vitamin E	0.1 mg
Riboflavin (B-2)	0.3 mg	Calcium	503.7 mg
Niacin	0.5 mg	Iron	0.2 mg
Vitamin B-6	0.1 mg	Phosphorus	248.6 mg
Vitamin B-12	0.9 µg	Magnesium	32.9 mg
Folate (total)	12.3 µg	Zinc	1.0 mg
Vitamin C	2.5 mg	Potassium	751.1 mg

Mocha Float

PER SERVING: 286.1 CALORIES — 3.5 g PROTEIN — 41.6 g CARBOHYDRATE — 0.7 g FIBER —
12.4 g TOTAL FAT — 7.6 g SATURATED FAT — 45.1 mg CHOLESTEROL — 71.6 mg SODIUM

$2/3$ cup strong coffee, cold

2 tablespoons chocolate syrup

Ice cubes

$1/2$ cup vanilla ice cream

Combine coffee and syrup in tall glass; stir to dissolve syrup. Add ice to glass; top with ice cream.

TIP: Garnish with whipped cream and chocolate curls, if you wish.

Makes 1 serving.

Nutritional Analysis per Serving

Vitamin A	137.3 RE	Vitamin D	0.0 µg
Thiamin (B-1)	0.0 mg	Vitamin E	0.0 mg
Riboflavin (B-2)	0.1 mg	Calcium	95.0 mg
Niacin	0.5 mg	Iron	0.9 mg
Vitamin B-6	0.0 mg	Phosphorus	120.3 mg
Vitamin B-12	0.3 µg	Magnesium	40.4 mg
Folate (total)	5.2 µg	Zinc	0.6 mg
Vitamin C	0.6 mg	Potassium	287.0 mg

Berry Nog

PER SERVING: 290.6 CALORIES — 13.8G PROTEIN — 61.2 g CARBOHYDRATE — 2.0 g FIBER —
0.9 g TOTAL FAT — 0.1 g SATURATED FAT — 3.1 mg CHOLESTEROL — 203.7 mg SODIUM

$^1/_2$ cup cholesterol-free real egg product

2 tablespoons honey

1 cup apricot nectar

$^2/_3$ cup orange juice

$^1/_2$ cup nonfat dry milk powder

1 tablespoon lemon juice

1 cup frozen strawberries, partially thawed

Process all ingredients in blender or food processor until smooth. Cover and chill. Stir well before serving.

Makes 2 servings.

NOTE: To avoid the risk of salmonella poisoning from raw eggs, pasteurized egg product has been used in this recipe.

Nutritional Analysis per Serving

Vitamin A	366.1 RE	Vitamin D	2.3 μg
Thiamin (B-1)	0.2 mg	Vitamin E	1.0 mg
Riboflavin (B-2)	1.4 mg	Calcium	254.2 mg
Niacin	1.0 mg	Iron	1.9 mg
Vitamin B-6	0.2 mg	Phosphorus	238.3 mg
Vitamin B-12	1.3 μg	Magnesium	40.6 mg
Folate (total)	68.2 μg	Zinc	1.6 mg
Vitamin C	58.7 mg	Potassium	710.9 mg

Tomato Refresher

PER SERVING: 98.3 CALORIES — 3.1 g PROTEIN — 23.9 g CARBOHYDRATE — 1.5 g FIBER —
0.4 g TOTAL FAT — 0 g SATURATED FAT — 0 mg CHOLESTEROL — 1,438.8 mg SODIUM

2 quarts tomato juice
2 cups orange juice
¼ cup lemon juice
1 teaspoon celery salt
1 tablespoon Worcestershire sauce
1 clove of garlic, minced

Combine all ingredients in large pitcher. Refrigerate, covered, for several hours.

Makes 6 servings.

Nutritional Analysis per Serving

Vitamin A	198.9 RE	Vitamin D	0.0 µg
Thiamin (B-1)	0.2 mg	Vitamin E	3.0 mg
Riboflavin (B-2)	0.1 mg	Calcium	42.0 mg
Niacin	2.5 mg	Iron	2.1 mg
Vitamin B-6	0.4 mg	Phosphorus	77.4 mg
Vitamin B-12	0.0 µg	Magnesium	45.6 mg
Folate (total)	91.2 µg	Zinc	0.5 mg
Vitamin C	105.7 mg	Potassium	904.3 mg

Apricot Tea Whirl

PER SERVING: 105.6 CALORIES — 2.5 g PROTEIN — 23.8 g CARBOHYDRATE — 0.8 g FIBER —
0.6 g TOTAL FAT — 0.3 g SATURATED FAT — 2.0 mg CHOLESTEROL — 31.3 mg SODIUM

1½ cups boiling water
6 cinnamon-apple herb tea bags
2 cans (12 ounces each) apricot nectar, chilled
1 cup low-fat vanilla yogurt
Ice cubes

Pour boiling water over tea bags in teapot or medium saucepan; let stand, covered 5 minutes. Remove tea bags; allow tea to cool. Process tea and remaining ingredients in blender or food processor until smooth. Serve over ice.

Makes 6 servings.

Nutritional Analysis per Serving

Vitamin A	171.0 RE	Vitamin D	0.0 µg
Thiamin (B-1)	0.0 mg	Vitamin E	0.1 mg
Riboflavin (B-2)	0.1 mg	Calcium	79.8 mg
Niacin	0.4 mg	Iron	0.6 mg
Vitamin B-6	0.0 mg	Phosphorus	66.4 mg
Vitamin B-12	0.2 µg	Magnesium	13.4 mg
Folate (total)	6.3 µg	Zinc	0.5 mg
Vitamin C	1.1 mg	Potassium	237.8 mg

Spiced Hot Chocolate

PER SERVING: 245.3 CALORIES — 9.1 g PROTEIN — 21.1 g CARBOHYDRATE — 2.5 g FIBER —
15.8 g TOTAL FAT — 9.3 g SATURATED FAT — 78.7 mg CHOLESTEROL — 183.1 mg SODIUM

2 ounces unsweetened chocolate

¼ cup water

3 cups whole milk

2–4 tablespoons packed light brown sugar*

⅛ teaspoon salt

1 teaspoon ground cinnamon

⅛ teaspoon ground allspice

⅛ teaspoon ground nutmeg

1 egg, lightly beaten

1 teaspoon vanilla

4 tablespoons reduced-fat whipped topping

Heat chocolate and water in medium saucepan over low heat until chocolate is melted, stirring constantly. Stir in milk, brown sugar, salt, and spices. Heat to simmering, stirring constantly. Whisk a small amount of milk mixture into egg; whisk egg mixture into saucepan. Add vanilla. Whisk constantly over low heat for 1 minute. Pour into cups or mugs; top with whipped topping. Makes 4 servings.

*Can substitute 4 packets of Equal

Nutritional Analysis per Serving

Vitamin A	82.2 RE	Vitamin D	2.0 µg
Thiamin (B-1)	0.1 mg	Vitamin E	0.5 mg
Riboflavin (B-2)	0.4 mg	Calcium	248.0 mg
Niacin	0.3 mg	Iron	1.5 mg
Vitamin B-6	0.1 mg	Phosphorus	253.8 mg
Vitamin B-12	0.8 µg	Magnesium	71.7 mg
Folate (total)	16.3 µg	Zinc	1.4 mg
Vitamin C	1.8 mg	Potassium	440.7 mg

Orange Sunrise

PER SERVING: 260.9 CALORIES — 13.7 g PROTEIN — 43.1 g CARBOHYDRATE — 0.2 g FIBER —
4.2 g TOTAL FAT — 2.6 g SATURATED FAT — 17.5 mg CHOLESTEROL — 198.4 mg SODIUM

$1/2$ cup cholesterol-free real egg product
$1/4$ cup frozen orange juice concentrate
2 tablespoons honey
2 cups 2% reduced-fat milk
1 carton (8 ounces) low-fat orange yogurt

Process egg product, orange juice, and honey in blender or food processor until smooth; add milk and yogurt. Blend until smooth and frothy.

Makes 3 servings.

NOTE: To avoid the risk of salmonella poisoning from raw eggs, pasteurized egg product has been used in this recipe.

Nutritional Analysis per Serving

Vitamin A	150.7 RE	Vitamin D	1.9 µg
Thiamin (B-1)	0.2 mg	Vitamin E	0.7 mg
Riboflavin (B-2)	1.1 mg	Calcium	348.0 mg
Niacin	0.5 mg	Iron	1.0 mg
Vitamin B-6	0.2 mg	Phosphorus	295.8 mg
Vitamin B-12	1.4 µg	Magnesium	45.9 mg
Folate (total)	74.0 µg	Zinc	1.7 mg
Vitamin C	34.9 mg	Potassium	637.3 mg

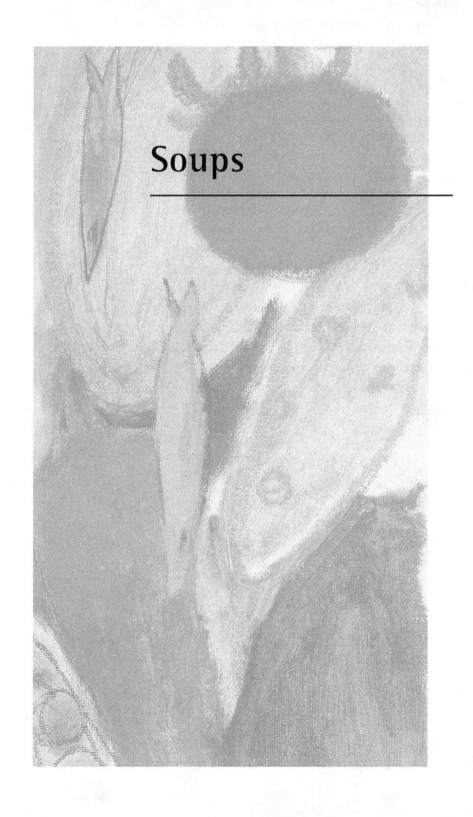

Soups

Catfish Soup

PER SERVING: 161.7 CALORIES — 22.4 g PROTEIN — 2.8 g CARBOHYDRATE — 0.3 g FIBER —
6.2 g TOTAL FAT — 2.4 g SATURATED FAT — 73.2 mg CHOLESTEROL — 266.0 mg SODIUM

1 onion, finely chopped
1 stalk of celery, finely chopped
1 tablespoon butter
2 pounds skinless catfish fillets, cut up
1 quart fish stock
1 cup 2% reduced-fat milk
Salt and pepper, to taste

Sauté onion and celery in butter in large saucepan until softened, about 5 minutes. Stir in fish, fish stock, and milk. Heat to
boiling; reduce heat and simmer, covered, until fish flakes easily.
Season to taste with salt and pepper.
    Serves 8.

Nutritional Analysis per Serving

Vitamin A	47.5 RE	Vitamin D	14.5 µg
Thiamin (B-1)	0.3 mg	Vitamin E	2.3 mg
Riboflavin (B-2)	0.2 mg	Calcium	61.8 mg
Niacin	3.6 mg	Iron	0.4 mg
Vitamin B-6	0.2 mg	Phosphorus	337.4 mg
Vitamin B-12	2.9 µg	Magnesium	40.5 mg
Folate (total)	39.7 µg	Zinc	0.8 mg
Vitamin C	2.3 mg	Potassium	657.1 mg

Mushroom–Clam Bisque

PER SERVING: 122.3 CALORIES — 12.6 g PROTEIN — 12.1 g CARBOHYDRATE — 1.2 g FIBER —
6.5 g TOTAL FAT — 3.9 g SATURATED FAT — 17.7 mg CHOLESTEROL — 853.0 mg SODIUM

10 ounces fresh mushrooms, finely chopped
2 tablespoons butter or margarine
1/4 cup all-purpose flour
2 bottles (8 ounces each) clam juice
1 cup fat-free milk
1 teaspoon dried thyme leaves
Salt and pepper, to taste

Sauté mushrooms in butter in medium saucepan until tender, about 5 minutes. Sprinkle sautéd mushrooms with flour and cook over medium heat, stirring frequently, until lightly browned, about 5 minutes. Stir in clam juice, milk, and thyme; heat to boiling. Reduce heat and simmer 15 minutes, stirring occasionally. Season to taste with salt and pepper.

Makes 4 servings.

Nutritional Analysis per Serving

Vitamin A	95.2 RE	Vitamin D	2.1 µg
Thiamin (B-1)	0.1 mg	Vitamin E	0.2 mg
Riboflavin (B-2)	0.4 mg	Calcium	88.5 mg
Niacin	3.4 mg	Iron	1.6 mg
Vitamin B-6	0.1 mg	Phosphorus	146.4 mg
Vitamin B-12	0.3 µg	Magnesium	16.5 mg
Folate (total)	24.8 µg	Zinc	0.8 mg
Vitamin C	2.4 mg	Potassium	377.1 mg

Mushroom–Shrimp Soup

PER SERVING: 378.2 CALORIES — 19.9 g PROTEIN — 33.7 g CARBOHYDRATE — 1.4 g FIBER —
17.8 g TOTAL FAT — 10.1 g SATURATED FAT — 162.6 mg CHOLESTEROL — 947.4 mg SODIUM

$1/4$ cup finely chopped onion

1 small potato, peeled, grated

1 tablespoon finely chopped chives

2 tablespoons butter or margarine

1 can ($10^3/4$ ounces) reduced-sodium, reduced-fat
cream of mushroom soup (condensed)

1 soup can 1% low-fat milk

4 ounces cooked, peeled, deveined shrimp, finely chopped

Salt and pepper, to taste

Sauté onion, potato, and chives in butter in medium saucepan until very tender. Stir in soup and milk, mixing well; heat to simmering and cook for 5 minutes. Stir in shrimp; simmer for an additional 3 minutes. Season to taste with salt and pepper.

Makes 2 servings.

Nutritional Analysis per Serving

Vitamin A	253.7 RE	Vitamin D	1.8 µg
Thiamin (B-1)	0.2 mg	Vitamin E	0.6 mg
Riboflavin (B-2)	0.4 mg	Calcium	364.2 mg
Niacin	2.9 mg	Iron	2.1 mg
Vitamin B-6	0.3 mg	Phosphorus	268.6 mg
Vitamin B-12	1.5 µg	Magnesium	56.5 mg
Folate (total)	21.4 µg	Zinc	1.7 mg
Vitamin C	9.2 mg	Potassium	1,143.3 mg

Cold Peach Soup

PER SERVING: 173.8 CALORIES — 5.1 g PROTEIN — 28.3 g CARBOHYDRATE — 2.6 g FIBER —
5.1 g TOTAL FAT — 3.0 g SATURATED FAT — 20.0 mg CHOLESTEROL — 40.5 mg SODIUM

5 large, ripe peaches, peeled, quartered
1/4 cup lemon juice
2 tablespoons frozen orange juice concentrate
2–3 tablespoons sugar*
1 cup reduced-fat sour cream
Ground nutmeg, as garnish

Process all ingredients, except nutmeg, in food processor or blender until smooth. Pour into medium bowl; refrigerate, covered, until well chilled. Serve soup in bowls; sprinkle with nutmeg.
Makes 4 servings.

*Can substitute 6 packets of Equal

Nutritional Analysis per Serving

Vitamin A	189.0 RE	Vitamin D	0.0 µg
Thiamin (B-1)	0.1 mg	Vitamin E	0.9 mg
Riboflavin (B-2)	0.2 mg	Calcium	130.1 mg
Niacin	1.3 mg	Iron	0.2 mg
Vitamin B-6	0.0 mg	Phosphorus	100.8 mg
Vitamin B-12	0.2 µg	Magnesium	12.5 mg
Folate (total)	19.4 µg	Zinc	0.2 mg
Vitamin C	27.3 mg	Potassium	460.2 mg

Two-Melon Soup

PER SERVING: 63.5 CALORIES — 1.2 g PROTEIN — 16.0 g CARBOHYDRATE — 1.3 g FIBER —
0.3 g TOTAL FAT — 0.1 g SATURATED FAT — 0 mg CHOLESTEROL — 16.7 mg SODIUM

1 small very ripe cantaloupe, peeled, seeded, cubed
1–2 tablespoons lemon juice
$1/2$ very ripe honeydew melon, peeled, seeded, cubed
2–3 tablespoons lime juice
$1 1/2$ teaspoons chopped fresh mint leaves
Fat-free sour cream, as garnish

Process cantaloupe and lemon juice in food processor or blender until very smooth; pour into medium bowl. Process honeydew and lime juice in food processor or blender until very smooth; pour into medium bowl. Refrigerate both mixtures, covered, for several hours or overnight. Using 2 ladles, pour equal amounts of both soups at the same time into chilled bowls; garnish with sour cream.

Makes 6 servings.

Nutritional Analysis per Serving

Vitamin A	300.2 RE	Vitamin D	0.0 µg
Thiamin (B-1)	0.1 mg	Vitamin E	0.3 mg
Riboflavin (B-2)	0.0 mg	Calcium	16.1 mg
Niacin	1.0 mg	Iron	0.3 mg
Vitamin B-6	0.2 mg	Phosphorus	24.6 mg
Vitamin B-12	0.0 µg	Magnesium	16.5 mg
Folate (total)	21.5 µg	Zinc	0.2 mg
Vitamin C	62.2 mg	Potassium	519.6 mg

Chicken Velvet Soup

PER SERVING: 246.3 CALORIES — 18.8 g PROTEIN — 11.6 g CARBOHYDRATE — 0.6 g FIBER —
13.5 g TOTAL FAT — 7.3 g SATURATED FAT — 78.9 mg CHOLESTEROL — 335.1 mg SODIUM

¹/₃ cup finely chopped green onions
2 tablespoons chopped parsley
1 tablespoon chopped fresh, or ¹/₂ teaspoon dried, tarragon leaves
3 tablespoons butter or margarine
¹/₃ cup all-purpose flour
1 cup whole milk
3 cups reduced-sodium, fat-free chicken broth
1 cup finely chopped cooked chicken breast
Salt and pepper, to taste

Sauté green onions, parsley, and tarragon in butter in medium
saucepan until tender, about 3 minutes. Blend in flour; cook
1 minute. Whisk in milk and chicken broth. Heat to boiling,
whisking frequently until thickened. Stir in chicken and season to
taste with salt and pepper.

Makes 4 servings.

Nutritional Analysis per Serving

Vitamin A	119.7 RE	Vitamin D	0.8 µg
Thiamin (B-1)	0.1 mg	Vitamin E	0.4 mg
Riboflavin (B-2)	0.2 mg	Calcium	92.1 mg
Niacin	3.7 mg	Iron	1.1 mg
Vitamin B-6	0.2 mg	Phosphorus	133.0 mg
Vitamin B-12	0.3 µg	Magnesium	22.1 mg
Folate (total)	28.6 µg	Zinc	0.7 mg
Vitamin C	4.7 mg	Potassium	211.1 mg

Tomato–Ham Soup

PER SERVING: 249.0 CALORIES — 21.8 g PROTEIN — 29.0 g CARBOHYDRATE — 2.8 g FIBER — 5.2 g TOTAL FAT — 4.3 g SATURATED FAT — 47.6 mg CHOLESTEROL — 2,065.4 mg SODIUM

1 can (10$^1/_2$ ounces) cream of tomato soup (condensed)
6 ounces smoked ham, very finely chopped
1 cup 2% milk
$^3/_4$–1 teaspoon dried basil leaves

Combine all ingredients in medium saucepan; heat over medium heat until hot, stirring frequently.

Makes 2 servings.

Nutritional Analysis per Serving

Vitamin A	138. RE	Vitamin D	1.2 µg
Thiamin (B-1)	0.1 mg	Vitamin E	0.1 mg
Riboflavin (B-2)	0.2 mg	Calcium	185.3 mg
Niacin	1.2 mg	Iron	1.9 mg
Vitamin B-6	0.1 mg	Phosphorus	118.5 mg
Vitamin B-12	0.4 µg	Magnesium	19.3 mg
Folate (total)	7.5 µg	Zinc	0.5 mg
Vitamin C	4.6 mg	Potassium	205.9 mg

Gazpacho de Madrid

PER SERVING: 137.8 CALORIES — 3.8 g PROTEIN — 22.1 g CARBOHYDRATE — 3.0 g FIBER —
4.8 g TOTAL FAT — 0.6 g SATURATED FAT — 0.2 mg CHOLESTEROL — 137.4 mg SODIUM

4 tomatoes, peeled, seeded, chopped

$^1/_3$ green bell pepper, cubed

$^1/_3$ cucumber, peeled, cubed

$^1/_4$ medium onion, chopped

2 garlic cloves

1$^1/_2$ cups reduced-sodium tomato juice

3 tablespoons red wine vinegar

1 tablespoon olive oil

2 cups fresh white bread crumbs, crusts removed, soaked in water until soft

Salt and pepper, to taste

Process tomatoes, bell pepper, cucumber, onion, and garlic in blender or food processor until finely chopped. Pour mixture into large bowl; stir in tomato juice, vinegar, oil, and the bread crumbs. Season to taste with salt and pepper. Refrigerate, covered, several hours or overnight.

Makes 4 servings.

Nutritional Analysis per Serving

Vitamin A	97.2 RE	Vitamin D	0.0 µg
Thiamin (B-1)	0.2 mg	Vitamin E	1.1 mg
Riboflavin (B-2)	0.1 mg	Calcium	42.4 mg
Niacin	1.8 mg	Iron	1.6 mg
Vitamin B-6	0.2 mg	Phosphorus	62.2 mg
Vitamin B-12	0.0 µg	Magnesium	23.7 mg
Folate (total)	46.6 µg	Zinc	0.3 mg
Vitamin C	43.0 mg	Potassium	370.3 mg

Orange-Scented Carrot Soup

PER SERVING: 189.5 CALORIES — 7.8 g PROTEIN — 23.6 g CARBOHYDRATE — 4.8 g FIBER —
7.6 g TOTAL FAT — 3.9 g SATURATED FAT — 35.2 mg CHOLESTEROL — 291.4 mg SODIUM

1 pound carrots, sliced

2 medium onions, chopped

2 tablespoons butter or margarine

2 tablespoons flour

3 cups reduced-sodium, fat-free chicken broth

$1/2$ cup orange juice

2 tablespoons lemon juice

1 tablespoon finely grated orange rind

$1/2$ teaspoon ground ginger

Salt and pepper, to taste

Sauté carrots and onions in butter in large saucepan until softened, about 5 minutes. Add flour and cook for 1 minute, stirring.
Add chicken broth, orange juice, lemon juice, orange rind, and
ginger. Heat to boiling; reduce heat and and simmer, covered, until
carrots are tender, about 30 minutes. Process in blender or food
processor until smooth; season to taste with salt and pepper.

Makes 4 servings.

Nutritional Analysis per Serving

Vitamin A	2,934.5 RE	Vitamin D	0.1 µg
Thiamin (B-1)	0.2 mg	Vitamin E	0.8 mg
Riboflavin (B-2)	0.1 mg	Calcium	50.6 mg
Niacin	1.5 mg	Iron	1.0 mg
Vitamin B-6	0.2 mg	Phosphorus	80.4 mg
Vitamin B-12	0.0 µg	Magnesium	28.1 mg
Folate (total)	40.2 µg	Zinc	0.4 mg
Vitamin C	32.5 mg	Potassium	536.4 mg

Garden Vegetable Soup

PER SERVING: 309.5 CALORIES — 15.1 g PROTEIN — 59.8 g CARBOHYDRATE — 11.5 g FIBER —
3.1 g TOTAL FAT — 0.9 g SATURATED FAT — 3.4 mg CHOLESTEROL — 369.2 mg SODIUM

1–2 slices bacon, chopped
2 onions, cubed
2 leeks, white parts only, sliced
1 parsnip, sliced
2 carrots, sliced
1 potato, cubed
3 cups reduced-sodium, fat-free beef broth
1 can (8 ounces) reduced-sodium tomatoes, undrained
2 bay leaves
1 teaspoon dried thyme leaves
1 tablespoon chopped parsley
Salt and pepper, to taste

Cook bacon in large saucepan over medium heat until crisp. Add the vegetables and sauté until lightly browned, about 8 minutes. Add remaining ingredients, except salt and pepper. Heat to boiling; reduce heat and simmer, covered, until vegetables are tender, about 20 minutes. Discard bay leaves. Process in blender or food processor until smooth; season to taste with salt and pepper.
Makes 2 servings.

Nutritional Analysis per Serving

Vitamin A	1,809.1 RE	Vitamin D	0.0 µg
Thiamin (B-1)	0.4 mg	Vitamin E	1.8 mg
Riboflavin (B-2)	0.2 mg	Calcium	175.6 mg
Niacin	3.6 mg	Iron	4.9 mg
Vitamin B-6	0.8 mg	Phosphorus	206.6 mg
Vitamin B-12	0.1 µg	Magnesium	95.6 mg
Folate (total)	152.0 µg	Zinc	1.4 mg
Vitamin C	58.9 mg	Potassium	1,297.4 mg

Autumn Bisque

PER SERVING: 218.0 CALORIES — 10.6 g PROTEIN — 32.9 g CARBOHYDRATE — 2.7 g FIBER —
5.8 g TOTAL FAT — 1.9 g SATURATED FAT — 85.7 mg CHOLESTEROL — 329.0 mg SODIUM

1 pound butternut squash, peeled, seeded, cubed

2 tart apples, peeled, cored, cubed

1 medium onion, chopped

2 slices bread, cubed

4 cups reduced-sodium, fat-free chicken broth

$1/2$ teaspoon dried rosemary leaves

$1/4$ teaspoon dried marjoram leaves

1–2 egg yolks

3–4 tablespoons light cream

Salt and pepper, to taste

Combine the squash, apples, onion, bread, chicken broth, and herbs in large saucepan. Heat to boiling; reduce heat and simmer, uncovered, 25 minutes or until squash and apples are tender. Process in blender or food processor until smooth. Return soup to saucepan; heat to boiling. Whisk egg yolks and cream in small bowl. Whisk small amount of hot soup into yolk mixture; whisk yolk mixture into saucepan. Whisk over low heat 1 minute; do not boil. Season to taste with salt and pepper.

Makes 4 servings.

Nutritional Analysis per Serving

Vitamin A	933.4 RE	Vitamin D	0.2 µg
Thiamin (B-1)	0.2 mg	Vitamin E	0.5 mg
Riboflavin (B-2)	0.1 mg	Calcium	97.4 mg
Niacin	2.0 mg	Iron	1.6 mg
Vitamin B-6	0.3 mg	Phosphorus	92.5 mg
Vitamin B-12	0.2 µg	Magnesium	49.6 mg
Folate (total)	56.6 µg	Zinc	0.5 mg
Vitamin C	29.7 mg	Potassium	556.2 mg

Quick Mushroom Soup

PER SERVING: 209.8 CALORIES — 14.1 g PROTEIN — 20.2 g CARBOHYDRATE — 1.3 g FIBER —
8.1 g TOTAL FAT — 4.0 g SATURATED FAT — 43.9 mg CHOLESTEROL — 381.1 mg SODIUM

1 cup finely chopped mushrooms

1 clove garlic, finely chopped

2 green onions, finely chopped

1 tablespoon butter or margarine

3 1/2 tablespoons flour

2 cups reduced-sodium, fat-free chicken broth

1 cup fat-free milk

1 tablespoon lemon juice

Salt and pepper, to taste

1 tablespoon parsley, finely chopped

Paprika, as garnish

Sauté mushrooms, garlic, and green onions in butter in medium saucepan until mushrooms are tender, about 5 minutes. Stir in flour; stir over medium heat for 1 minute. Stir in chicken broth and milk; heat to boiling, stirring constantly. Reduce heat and simmer, uncovered, 5 minutes. Stir in lemon juice; season to taste with salt and pepper. Stir in parsley; spoon into bowls and sprinkle with paprika.

Makes 2 servings.

Nutritional Analysis per Serving

Vitamin A	147.2 RE	Vitamin D	2.0 µg
Thiamin (B-1)	0.2 mg	Vitamin E	0.3 mg
Riboflavin (B-2)	0.4 mg	Calcium	172.9 mg
Niacin	2.5 mg	Iron	1.4 mg
Vitamin B-6	0.1 mg	Phosphorus	186.0 mg
Vitamin B-12	0.5 µg	Magnesium	24.9 mg
Folate (total)	45.1 µg	Zinc	0.9 mg
Vitamin C	11.4 mg	Potassium	416.8 mg

Leek and Potato Soup

PER SERVING: 233.1 CALORIES — 9.6 g PROTEIN — 36.7 g CARBOHYDRATE — 3.2 g FIBER —
5.4 g TOTAL FAT — 2.6 g SATURATED FAT — 27.6 mg CHOLESTEROL — 255.3 mg SODIUM

6 leeks, white parts only, thinly sliced
2 tablespoons butter
4 potatoes, peeled, sliced
1 quart reduced-sodium, fat-free chicken broth
3/4 cup fat-free sour cream
Salt and pepper, to taste
Ground nutmeg, to taste

Sauté leeks in butter in large saucepan until softened, about
8 minutes. Add potatoes and chicken broth. Heat to boiling;
reduce heat and simmer, covered, until potatoes are tender, about
30 minutes. Process in blender or food processor until smooth.
Return to saucepan; heat to simmer. Whisk in sour cream. Season
to taste with salt, pepper, and nutmeg.

Makes 6 servings.

Nutritional Analysis per Serving

Vitamin A	106.6 RE	Vitamin D	0.1 µg
Thiamin (B-1)	0.4 mg	Vitamin E	0.9 mg
Riboflavin (B-2)	0.1 mg	Calcium	101.0 mg
Niacin	1.5 mg	Iron	2.2 mg
Vitamin B-6	0.5 mg	Phosphorus	108.6 mg
Vitamin B-12	0.1 µg	Magnesium	43.2 mg
Folate (total)	65.3 µg	Zinc	0.4 mg
Vitamin C	17.4 mg	Potassium	528.9 mg

Potato and Turnip Soup

PER SERVING: 196.8 CALORIES — 15.5 g PROTEIN — 27.5 g CARBOHYDRATE — 3.4 g FIBER —
2.7 g TOTAL FAT — 0.9 g SATURATED FAT — 28.2 mg CHOLESTEROL — 304.6 mg SODIUM

3 large potatoes, peeled, cubed
2 large turnips, peeled, cubed
1 large onion, chopped
3 cups reduced-sodium, fat-free chicken or vegetable broth
1 cup (4 ounces) shredded, reduced-fat Swiss cheese
Salt and pepper, to taste

Combine potatoes, turnips, onion, and broth in large saucepan. Heat to boiling; reduce heat and simmer, covered, until vegetables are tender. Process in blender or food processor until smooth; return soup to saucepan. Heat to boiling; reduce heat and stir in cheese, stirring over low heat until melted. Season to taste with salt and pepper.

Makes 4 servings.

Nutritional Analysis per Serving

Vitamin A	17.6 RE	Vitamin D	0.0 µg
Thiamin (B-1)	0.1 mg	Vitamin E	0.2 mg
Riboflavin (B-2)	0.1 mg	Calcium	291.9 mg
Niacin	1.6 mg	Iron	0.6 mg
Vitamin B-6	0.4 mg	Phosphorus	230.0 mg
Vitamin B-12	0.5 µg	Magnesium	39.6 mg
Folate (total)	25.2 µg	Zinc	1.5 mg
Vitamin C	22.1 mg	Potassium	524.3 mg

Cheddar Chowder

PER SERVING: 200.2 CALORIES — 11.5 g PROTEIN — 14.0 g CARBOHYDRATE — 0.8 g FIBER —
10.8 g TOTAL FAT — 6.4 g SATURATED FAT — 43.0 mg CHOLESTEROL — 290.9 mg SODIUM

1/4 cup finely chopped onion

1/4 cup finely chopped carrot

1/4 cup finely chopped celery

1 tablespoon butter or margarine

1/4 cup all-purpose flour

2 cups 2% reduced-fat milk

1 can (13 3/4 ounces) reduced-sodium, fat-free chicken broth

1/2 cup (2 ounces) shredded sharp Cheddar cheese

1/4 teaspoon paprika

Salt and pepper, to taste

Sauté onion, carrot, and celery in butter in medium saucepan until tender, about 5 minutes. Stir in flour; cook 1 minute. Stir in milk and chicken broth. Heat to boiling; reduce heat and simmer, covered, 10 minutes. Stir in cheese, stirring over low heat until melted. Stir in paprika; season to taste with salt and pepper.

Makes 4 servings.

Nutritional Analysis per Serving

Vitamin A	359.4 RE	Vitamin D	1.3 µg
Thiamin (B-1)	0.1 mg	Vitamin E	0.3 mg
Riboflavin (B-2)	0.3 mg	Calcium	260.0 mg
Niacin	0.7 mg	Iron	0.6 mg
Vitamin B-6	0.1 mg	Phosphorus	206.5 mg
Vitamin B-12	0.6 µg	Magnesium	26.0 mg
Folate (total)	26.0 µg	Zinc	1.0 mg
Vitamin C	3.2 mg	Potassium	275.9 mg

Cheddar–Asparagus Soup

PER SERVING: 199.3 CALORIES — 12.6 g PROTEIN — 14.6 g CARBOHYDRATE — 2.5 g FIBER —
9.1 g TOTAL FAT — 4.5 g SATURATED FAT — 45.8 mg CHOLESTEROL — 365.5 mg SODIUM

³/₄ cup finely chopped onion
³/₄ cup finely chopped celery
¹/₂ teaspoon dry mustard
2 tablespoons butter or margarine
6 cups fat-free, reduced-sodium chicken broth, divided
1 pound asparagus, trimmed, cut into 1-inch pieces
¹/₄ cup dry sherry
¹/₂ teaspoon crumbled bay leaf
Dash hot pepper sauce
Dash worcestershire sauce
¹/₂ cup all-purpose flour
¹/₂ cup (4 ounces) shredded mild Cheddar cheese

Sauté onion, celery, and dry mustard in butter in large saucepan until vegetables are tender, about 5 minutes. Stir in 5 cups
chicken broth; heat to boiling. Stir in remaining ingredients,
except flour and cheese. Reduce heat and simmer, covered, until
asparagus is tender, about 20 minutes. Process soup in blender or
food processor until smooth. Return soup to saucepan and heat
to boiling; stir in combined flour and remaining 1 cup broth.
Simmer until thickened, stirring constantly. Add cheese and stir
until melted.

Makes 6 servings.

Nutritional Analysis per Serving

Vitamin A	110.0 RE	Vitamin D	0.1 µg
Thiamin (B-1)	0.2 mg	Vitamin E	1.7 mg
Riboflavin (B-2)	0.2 mg	Calcium	98.2 mg
Niacin	1.6 mg	Iron	1.4 mg
Vitamin B-6	0.2 mg	Phosphorus	114.8 mg
Vitamin B-12	0.1 µg	Magnesium	23.3 mg
Folate (total)	122.9 µg	Zinc	0.8 mg
Vitamin C	12.3 mg	Potassium	311.6 mg

Guacamole Soup

PER SERVING: 219.6 CALORIES — 8.5 g PROTEIN — 14.5 g CARBOHYDRATE — 5.6 g FIBER —
15.5 g TOTAL FAT — 2.3 g SATURATED FAT — 11.4 mg CHOLESTEROL — 265.9 mg SODIUM

1 can (13³/₄ ounces) reduced-sodium, fat-free chicken broth
2 medium avocados, seeded, peeled, cubed
1 large tomato, peeled, seeded, chopped
1 can (4 ounces) chopped green chilies
¹/₄ cup chopped onion
2 tablespoons lemon juice
1 cup fat-free plain yogurt
Salt and pepper, to taste

Process all ingredients, except salt and pepper, in a blender or
food processor until smooth. Pour into bowl and season to taste
with salt and pepper. Refrigerate, covered, until well chilled.
Makes 4 servings.

Nutritional Analysis per Serving

Vitamin A	72.2 RE	Vitamin D	0.0 µg
Thiamin (B-1)	0.1 mg	Vitamin E	1.3 mg
Riboflavin (B-2)	0.3 mg	Calcium	173.1 mg
Niacin	1.9 mg	Iron	1.2 mg
Vitamin B-6	0.3 mg	Phosphorus	142.9 mg
Vitamin B-12	0.4 µg	Magnesium	51.2 mg
Folate (total)	70.8 µg	Zinc	1.0 mg
Vitamin C	22.9 mg	Potassium	787.3 mg

Acorn Squash Soup

PER SERVING: 149.0 CALORIES — 8.3 g PROTEIN — 21.5 g CARBOHYDRATE — 3.0 g FIBER —
4.2 g TOTAL FAT — 1.7 g SATURATED FAT — 29.2 mg CHOLESTEROL — 271.1 mg SODIUM

2 pounds acorn squash, halved, seeded
2 large leeks, white parts only, sliced
1 tablespoon butter
5 cups reduced-sodium, fat-free chicken broth
1 tablespoon tomato paste
1 large thyme sprig, or $^1/_2$ teaspoon dried thyme leaves
Salt and white pepper, to taste
$^1/_2$ cup whole milk or light cream

Arrange squash cut sides down in roasting pan. Add $^1/_2$ inch water. Bake covered at 325 degrees until squash is tender, about 30 minutes. Sauté leeks in butter in large saucepan until tender, about 5 minutes. Scoop out squash pulp and add to leeks. Stir in chicken broth, tomato paste, and thyme. Heat to boiling; reduce heat and simmer until squash is very soft, about 20 minutes. Discard thyme. Process soup in blender or food processor until smooth. Return soup to saucepan; heat to boiling. Season to taste with salt and white pepper. Stir in milk.

Makes 6 servings.

Nutritional Analysis per Serving

Vitamin A	86.6 RE	Vitamin D	0.2 µg
Thiamin (B-1)	0.2 mg	Vitamin E	0.5 mg
Riboflavin (B-2)	0.1 mg	Calcium	95.4 mg
Niacin	1.3 mg	Iron	1.9 mg
Vitamin B-6	0.3 mg	Phosphorus	86.7 mg
Vitamin B-12	0.1 µg	Magnesium	61.0 mg
Folate (total)	46.7 µg	Zinc	0.3 mg
Vitamin C	21.6 mg	Potassium	636.2 mg

Sweet Pepper Soup

PER SERVING: 99.6 CALORIES — 8.5 g PROTEIN — 12.8 g CARBOHYDRATE — 2.9 g FIBER —
1.8 g TOTAL FAT — 0.1 g SATURATED FAT — 25.0 mg CHOLESTEROL — 253.9 mg SODIUM

5 medium red, yellow, or green bell peppers, seeded, cut into 1-inch cubes
1 medium red onion, cut into 1-inch chunks
1 medium potato, peeled, cut into 1-inch cubes
6 cups reduced-sodium, fat-free chicken broth
3 bay leaves
1/2 teaspoon dried thyme leaves
1 whole clove
Salt and pepper, to taste

Combine all ingredients, except salt and pepper, in large saucepan; heat to boiling. Reduce heat and simmer, covered, until vegetables are tender, about 30 minutes. Discard clove. Process soup in blender or food processor until smooth; season to taste with salt and pepper. Serve hot or cold.

Makes 6 servings.

Nutritional Analysis per Serving

Vitamin A	567.6 RE	Vitamin D	0.0 µg
Thiamin (B-1)	0.1 mg	Vitamin E	0.7 mg
Riboflavin (B-2)	0.0 mg	Calcium	19.4 mg
Niacin	0.8 mg	Iron	0.8 mg
Vitamin B-6	0.3 mg	Phosphorus	34.6 mg
Vitamin B-12	0.0 µg	Magnesium	17.0 mg
Folate (total)	28.2 µg	Zinc	0.2 mg
Vitamin C	191.5 mg	Potassium	281.7 mg

Cold Broccoli Soup

PER SERVING: 138.1 CALORIES — 9.1 g PROTEIN — 20.4 g CARBOHYDRATE — 2.2 g FIBER —
2.0 g TOTAL FAT — 1.1 g SATURATED FAT — 7.3 mg CHOLESTEROL — 492.8 mg SODIUM

1 package (10 ounces) frozen chopped broccoli, partially thawed
1 1/2 cups 2% reduced-fat milk, divided
1 cup fat-free sour cream
1 teaspoon instant minced onion
2 teaspoons beef bouillon crystals
Salt and pepper, to taste
Dash ground nutmeg

Process broccoli, milk, sour cream, onion, and bouillon crystals in blender or food processor until smooth. Pour into medium bowl. Season to taste with salt, pepper, and nutmeg. Refrigerate, covered, until cold.

Makes 4 servings.

Nutritional Analysis per Serving

Vitamin A	318.9 RE	Vitamin D	0.9 µg
Thiamin (B-1)	0.1 mg	Vitamin E	1.1 mg
Riboflavin (B-2)	0.4 mg	Calcium	232.4 mg
Niacin	0.4 mg	Iron	0.6 mg
Vitamin B-6	0.1 mg	Phosphorus	203.6 mg
Vitamin B-12	0.6 µg	Magnesium	26.8 mg
Folate (total)	52.8 µg	Zinc	0.7 mg
Vitamin C	41.2 mg	Potassium	451.8 mg

Chilled Spanish Tomato Soup

PER SERVING: 206.2 CALORIES — 7.8 g PROTEIN — 27.1 g CARBOHYDRATE — 4.9 g FIBER —
8.9 g TOTAL FAT — 1.1 g SATURATED FAT — 12.6 mg CHOLESTEROL — 215.9 mg SODIUM

1 pound tomatoes, peeled, seeded

1 onion, cubed

1 green bell pepper, cubed

1 clove garlic

1–2 tablespoons olive oil

2 tablespoons lemon juice

1 tablespoon red wine vinegar

1 slice white bread

1 cup fat-free, reduced-sodium chicken broth

Salt and pepper, to taste

Process all ingredients, except salt and pepper, in blender until smooth. Refrigerate, covered, several hours or overnight; season to taste with salt and pepper.

Makes 2 servings.

Nutritional Analysis per Serving

Vitamin A	178.4 RE	Vitamin D	0.0 µg
Thiamin (B-1)	0.3 mg	Vitamin E	2.2 mg
Riboflavin (B-2)	0.2 mg	Calcium	45.0 mg
Niacin	2.3 mg	Iron	1.9 mg
Vitamin B-6	0.4 mg	Phosphorus	98.9 mg
Vitamin B-12	0.0 µg	Magnesium	40.7 mg
Folate (total)	71.5 µg	Zinc	0.5 mg
Vitamin C	107.5 mg	Potassium	735.0 mg

Chilled Asparagus Soup

PER SERVING: 127.9 CALORIES — 8.3 g PROTEIN — 14.9 g CARBOHYDRATE — 1.4 g FIBER —
4.2 g TOTAL FAT — 2.6 g SATURATED FAT — 17.1 mg CHOLESTEROL — 90.5 mg SODIUM

1 package (10 ounces) frozen cut asparagus, cooked, drained
2 cups whole milk, divided
1/2 cup fat-free sour cream
1 teaspoon instant minced onion
Salt and pepper, to taste

Process all ingredients, except salt and pepper, in blender or
food processor until smooth. Pour into medium bowl. Refrigerate,
covered, several hours or until chilled. Season to taste with salt
and pepper.

Makes 4 servings.

Nutritional Analysis per Serving

Vitamin A	165.2 RE	Vitamin D	1.2 µg
Thiamin (B-1)	0.1 mg	Vitamin E	1.7 mg
Riboflavin (B-2)	0.4 mg	Calcium	204.0 mg
Niacin	1.0 mg	Iron	0.6 mg
Vitamin B-6	0.1 mg	Phosphorus	200.1 mg
Vitamin B-12	1.0 µg	Magnesium	26.2 mg
Folate (total)	142.2 µg	Zinc	0.9 mg
Vitamin C	23.9 mg	Potassium	441.5 mg

Creamy Cold Avocado Soup

PER SERVING: 311.2 CALORIES — 8.6 g PROTEIN — 17.8 g CARBOHYDRATE — 4.5 g FIBER —
23.8 g TOTAL FAT — 6.3 g SATURATED FAT — 28.9 mg CHOLESTEROL — 231.6 mg SODIUM

3 tablespoons butter or margarine

3 tablespoons flour

3 cups reduced-sodium, fat-free chicken broth

3 avocados, peeled, pitted

1 cup fat-free sour cream

1 1/2 teaspoons lemon juice

1/2 teaspoon ground white pepper

2 scallions, minced

1/2 small hot red chili, minced, or 1/4 teaspoon cayenne pepper

1 tablespoon olive oil

Melt butter in medium saucepan over low heat. Whisk in flour until smooth, and cook 2 minutes, whisking constantly; do not brown. Whisk in chicken broth; heat to boiling, whisking frequently. Reduce heat and simmer, uncovered, 5 minutes. Cool. Process avocados, sour cream, and half the chicken broth mixture in blender or food processor until smooth. Pour into medium bowl. Whisk in remaining chicken broth mixture, lemon juice, and white pepper. Refrigerate, covered, until chilled, about 3 hours.

Combine remaining ingredients in small bowl. To serve, divide the soup among 6 bowls and spoon scallion-pepper mixture into the center of each.

Makes 6 servings.

Nutritional Analysis per Serving

Vitamin A	230.6 RE	Vitamin D	0.1 µg
Thiamin (B-1)	0.1 mg	Vitamin E	1.6 mg
Riboflavin (B-2)	0.2 mg	Calcium	69.9 mg
Niacin	1.9 mg	Iron	1.4 mg
Vitamin B-6	0.3 mg	Phosphorus	98.9 mg
Vitamin B-12	0.2 µg	Magnesium	38.0 mg
Folate (total)	66.5 µg	Zinc	0.4 mg
Vitamin C	17.4 mg	Potassium	665.4 mg

Cauliflower Soup

PER SERVING: 254.6 CALORIES — 15.2 g PROTEIN — 17.3 g CARBOHYDRATE — 6.3 g FIBER —
15.0 g TOTAL FAT — 8.2 g SATURATED FAT — 62.0 mg CHOLESTEROL — 436.6 mg SODIUM

$^2/_3$ cup finely chopped onion
3 tablespoons butter or margarine
2 tablespoons flour
2 cans (13$^3/_4$ ounces each) reduced-sodium, fat-free chicken broth
2 cups whole milk
$^1/_2$ tablespoon Worcestershire sauce
1 medium head cauliflower, finely chopped, cooked
Salt and pepper, to taste
Chopped parsley, as garnish

Sauté onion in butter in large saucepan until tender, about
5 minutes. Stir in flour; cook, stirring, 1 minute. Add chicken
broth and heat to boiling, stirring constantly. Stir in milk, Worcestershire sauce, and cauliflower. Heat to boiling; reduce heat and
simmer for 2 minutes. Season to taste with salt and pepper;
sprinkle with parsley.

Makes 4 servings.

Nutritional Analysis per Serving

Vitamin A	126.6 RE	Vitamin D	1.4 µg
Thiamin (B-1)	0.2 mg	Vitamin E	0.3 mg
Riboflavin (B-2)	0.4 mg	Calcium	201.8 mg
Niacin	1.6 mg	Iron	1.3 mg
Vitamin B-6	0.6 mg	Phosphorus	232.2 mg
Vitamin B-12	0.5 µg	Magnesium	56.6 mg
Folate (total)	17.7 µg	Zinc	1.2 mg
Vitamin C	151.8 mg	Potassium	894.8 mg

Curried Pumpkin Soup

PER SERVING: 151.3 CALORIES — 7.1 g PROTEIN — 14.5 g CARBOHYDRATE — 3.0 g FIBER —
7.8 g TOTAL FAT — 4.4 g SATURATED FAT — 32.8 mg CHOLESTEROL — 190.4 mg SODIUM

1 large onion, finely chopped

1 clove garlic, minced

2 teaspoons curry powder

2 tablespoons butter or margarine

2 tablespoons flour

2¹/₂ cups reduced-sodium, fat-free chicken broth

2 cups whole milk, or half-and-half

2 cups canned pumpkin

Salt and pepper, to taste

Sauté onion, garlic, and curry powder in butter in large sauce-pan until soft, about 5 minutes. Stir in flour and cook 1 minute. Add chicken broth, milk, and pumpkin. Heat to boiling; reduce heat and simmer, covered, 10 minutes. Season to taste with salt and pepper.

Makes 6 servings.

Nutritional Analysis per Serving

Vitamin A	1,865.1 RE	Vitamin D	0.9 µg
Thiamin (B-1)	0.1 mg	Vitamin E	1.1 mg
Riboflavin (B-2)	0.2 mg	Calcium	127.4 mg
Niacin	0.6 mg	Iron	1.6 mg
Vitamin B-6	0.1 mg	Phosphorus	117.3 mg
Vitamin B-12	0.3 µg	Magnesium	33.7 mg
Folate (total)	22.6 µg	Zinc	0.5 mg
Vitamin C	5.6 mg	Potassium	337.0 mg

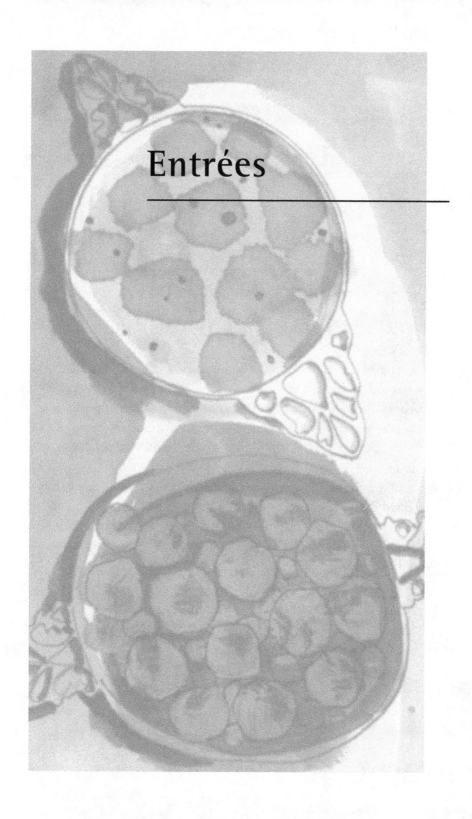

Entrées

Salmon Tetrazzini

PER SERVING: 404.2 CALORIES — 31.8 g PROTEIN — 30.6 g CARBOHYDRATE — 1.8 g FIBER —
16.4 g TOTAL FAT — 7.9 g SATURATED FAT — 72.7 mg CHOLESTEROL — 804.9 mg SODIUM

1 can (15 ounces) salmon
$1^1/_2$–2 cups whole milk
2 tablespoons butter or margarine, melted
2 tablespoons flour
Salt and pepper, to taste
Dash nutmeg
2 cups cooked spaghetti, finely chopped
1 can (4 ounces) mushrooms, drained, finely chopped
2 tablespoons grated Parmesan cheese
2 tablespoons unseasoned dry bread crumbs

To prepare sauce, drain salmon, reserving liquid; discard bones and skin. Add enough milk to reserved liquid to measure 2 cups. Combine butter and flour in medium saucepan; cook over medium heat 1 minute. Stir in milk mixture gradually; heat to boiling, stirring constantly. Season to taste with salt, pepper, and nutmeg.

Mix half the sauce with spaghetti and mushrooms in a lightly greased 2-quart casserole. Stir salmon into remaining sauce and spoon salmon and sauce mixture into center of spaghetti; sprinkle with cheese and crumbs. Bake at 350 degrees for 30 minutes or until bubbly.

Makes 4 servings.

Nutritional Analysis per Serving

Vitamin A	108.4 RE	Vitamin D	7.0 µg
Thiamin (B-1)	0.3 mg	Vitamin E	2.0 mg
Riboflavin (B-2)	0.4 mg	Calcium	423.0 mg
Niacin	9.2 mg	Iron	2.3 mg
Vitamin B-6	0.5 mg	Phosphorus	530.3 mg
Vitamin B-12	5.1 µg	Magnesium	60.2 mg
Folate (total)	85.0 µg	Zinc	1.9 mg
Vitamin C	0.8 mg	Potassium	496.0 mg

Salmon Quiche

PER SERVING: 441.0 CALORIES — 32.9 g PROTEIN — 22.1 g CARBOHYDRATE — 0.7 g FIBER — 23.9 g TOTAL FAT — 8.6 g SATURATED FAT — 196.8 mg CHOLESTEROL — 880.4 mg SODIUM

$^1/_2$ medium onion, finely chopped

1 teaspoon butter or margarine

2 cans (5.33 ounces each) evaporated milk

4 eggs, beaten

1 can (15 ounces) salmon, drained, bones and skin discarded

1$^1/_2$ cups (6 ounces) shredded reduced-fat Swiss cheese

$^1/_2$ teaspoon salt

$^1/_2$ teaspoon pepper

1 unbaked 9-inch pie shell

Sauté onion in butter in medium skillet until tender, about 4 minutes. Add evaporated milk, eggs, salmon, cheese, and salt and pepper, mixing well. Pour into pie shell and bake at 375 degrees until set and sharp knife inserted halfway between center and edge comes out clean, about 40 minutes.

Makes 6 servings.

Nutritional Analysis per Serving

Vitamin A	130.5 RE	Vitamin D	5.5 µg
Thiamin (B-1)	0.2 mg	Vitamin E	1.6 mg
Riboflavin (B-2)	0.6 mg	Calcium	604.7 mg
Niacin	6.1 mg	Iron	2.1 mg
Vitamin B-6	0.4 mg	Phosphorus	611.1 mg
Vitamin B-12	4.0 µg	Magnesium	53.2 mg
Folate (total)	57.8 µg	Zinc	2.7 mg
Vitamin C	1.7 mg	Potassium	489.5 mg

Baked Crab Casserole

PER SERVING: 315.5 CALORIES — 33.8 g PROTEIN — 19.2 g CARBOHYDRATE — 0.9 g FIBER — 9.8 g TOTAL FAT — 4.6 g SATURATED FAT — 152.6 mg CHOLESTEROL — 1,164.1 mg SODIUM

$1/2$ cup minced green onions

2 tablespoons butter or margarine

$1/4$ cup all-purpose flour

2 cups fat-free milk

$1/4$ teaspoon pepper

$1/2$ teaspoon celery salt

1 egg yolk, lightly beaten

2 tablespoons dry sherry

1 cup fresh white bread crumbs, divided

1 pound crabmeat

1 tablespoon chopped parsley

Paprika, as garnish

Sauté green onions in butter in medium saucepan until tender, about 3 minutes. Stir in flour and cook 1 minute. Whisk in milk, pepper, and celery salt; heat to boiling over medium heat, whisking constantly. Remove from heat; whisk in egg yolk. Stir in sherry, $3/4$ cup bread crumbs, crabmeat, and parsley. Spoon into greased $1^{1}/2$-quart casserole. Top with remaining $1/4$ cup bread crumbs. Sprinkle with paprika. Bake uncovered at 400 degrees 25 minutes, or until hot and bubbly.

Makes 4 servings.

Nutritional Analysis per Serving

Vitamin A	224.3 RE	Vitamin D	1.5 µg
Thiamin (B-1)	0.3 mg	Vitamin E	0.4 mg
Riboflavin (B-2)	0.6 mg	Calcium	220.4 mg
Niacin	4.4 mg	Iron	4.5 mg
Vitamin B-6	0.3 mg	Phosphorus	316.2 mg
Vitamin B-12	12.4 µg	Magnesium	93.8 mg
Folate (total)	92.3 µg	Zinc	4.9 mg
Vitamin C	13.0 mg	Potassium	506.3 mg

Creamy Shrimp and Noodles

PER SERVING: 409.3 CALORIES — 33.0 g PROTEIN — 36.4 g CARBOHYDRATE — 2.3 g FIBER —
14.1 g TOTAL FAT — 7.1 g SATURATED FAT — 242.7 mg CHOLESTEROL — 321.7 mg SODIUM

1 cup finely chopped onion
^{1}/$_2$ cup finely chopped green bell pepper
1 tablespoon butter or margarine
1 cup finely chopped, drained, canned tomatoes
1 tablespoon paprika
1 cup reduced-fat sour cream
1 package (3 ounces) cream cheese, cubed
1^1/$_2$ pounds peeled deveined shrimp, cooked, finely chopped
1 package (8 ounces) thin egg noodles, cooked, drained, chopped
Salt and pepper, to taste

Sauté onion and bell pepper in butter in large skillet until softened, about 5 minutes, stirring occasionally. Stir in tomatoes and
paprika; heat to boiling. Reduce heat and simmer until thickened,
about 5 minutes. Add sour cream and cream cheese, stirring over
medium heat until cream cheese is melted. Do not boil. Stir in
shrimp and noodles; heat over medium heat until heated through.
Season to taste with salt and pepper.

Makes 6 servings.

Nutritional Analysis per Serving

Vitamin A	310.0 RE	Vitamin D	4.3 µg
Thiamin (B-1)	0.3 mg	Vitamin E	1.4 mg
Riboflavin (B-2)	0.3 mg	Calcium	182.4 mg
Niacin	5.3 mg	Iron	4.8 mg
Vitamin B-6	0.3 mg	Phosphorus	369.1 mg
Vitamin B-12	1.6 µg	Magnesium	72.8 mg
Folate (total)	77.8 µg	Zinc	2.1 mg
Vitamin C	21.0 mg	Potassium	524.1 mg

Shrimp and Rice Casserole

PER SERVING: 295.1 CALORIES — 26.1 g PROTEIN — 26.8 g CARBOHYDRATE — 1.3 g FIBER —
8.2 g TOTAL FAT — 3.2 g SATURATED FAT — 183.1 mg CHOLESTEROL — 774.1 mg SODIUM

1 green bell pepper, finely chopped

1 onion, finely chopped

1 tablespoon butter

2 cups cooked rice

1 can (10³/₄ ounces) low-sodium, reduced-fat cream of mushroom soup (condensed)

1 can (10³/₄ ounces), cream of celery soup (condensed)

1¹/₂ pounds peeled shrimp, cooked, finely chopped

Cayenne pepper, to taste

Sauté bell pepper and onion in butter in medium saucepan until tender, about 8 minutes. Stir in rice, soups, and shrimp. Season to taste with cayenne pepper. Spoon into lightly greased 13 x 9-inch baking dish. Bake at 350 degrees, uncovered, until lightly browned, about 45 minutes.

Makes 6 servings.

Nutritional Analysis per Serving

Vitamin A	111.9 RE	Vitamin D	4.3 µg
Thiamin (B-1)	0.1 mg	Vitamin E	1.2 mg
Riboflavin (B-2)	0.1 mg	Calcium	121.1 mg
Niacin	3.8 mg	Iron	3.7 mg
Vitamin B-6	0.2 mg	Phosphorus	242.3 mg
Vitamin B-12	1.2 µg	Magnesium	52.1 mg
Folate (total)	41.0 µg	Zinc	1.6 mg
Vitamin C	20.7 mg	Potassium	479.0 mg

Imperial Creamed Crab

PER SERVING: 163.9 CALORIES — 19.2 g PROTEIN — 6.6 g CARBOHYDRATE — 0.3 g FIBER —
6.1 g TOTAL FAT — 3.3 g SATURATED FAT — 54.4 mg CHOLESTEROL — 1,010.8 mg SODIUM

1 pound crabmeat, flaked, or cooked shrimp, finely chopped
2 tablespoons lemon juice
$^1/_2$ package (8-ounce size) reduced-fat cream cheese, softened
$^1/_2$ cup whole milk, or light cream
3 green onions, finely chopped
$^1/_2$ teaspoon dry dill weed
Salt and pepper, to taste
$^1/_4$ cup grated Parmesan cheese
$^1/_4$ cup seasoned dry bread crumbs

Mix crabmeat, lemon juice, cream cheese, milk, green onions, and dill weed in medium bowl. Season to taste with salt and pepper. Spoon into lightly greased 1-quart casserole. Sprinkle with combined cheese and bread crumbs. Bake uncovered at 350 degrees until hot through, about 20 minutes.

Makes 6 servings.

Serve over a baked potato or with steamed rice.**

**Nutritional information does not include the potato or rice accompaniment

Nutritional Analysis per Serving

Vitamin A	69.6 RE	Vitamin D	0.2 µg
Thiamin (B-1)	0.1 mg	Vitamin E	1.2 mg
Riboflavin (B-2)	0.1 mg	Calcium	155.7 mg
Niacin	1.4 mg	Iron	1.0 mg
Vitamin B-6	0.2 mg	Phosphorus	291.1 mg
Vitamin B-12	8.8 µg	Magnesium	56.2 mg
Folate (total)	52.8 µg	Zinc	6.0 mg
Vitamin C	9.7 mg	Potassium	304.6 mg

Hot Crab and Avocado Casserole

PER SERVING: 302.2 CALORIES — 22.9 g PROTEIN — 12.8 g CARBOHYDRATE — 3.3 g FIBER —
18.5 g TOTAL FAT — 6.5 g SATURATED FAT — 93.5 mg CHOLESTEROL — 429.1 mg SODIUM

$1/3$ cup chopped onion

$1/3$ cup chopped red bell pepper

1 teaspoon dried thyme leaves

2 tablespoons butter or margarine

3 tablespoons flour

2 cups 2% reduced-fat milk

3 cans ($5^1/2$ ounces each) crabmeat, drained, flaked

2 small avocados, peeled, pitted, chopped

2 tablespoons lemon juice

Salt and cayenne pepper, to taste

$1/2$ cup (2 ounces) shredded reduced-fat Monterey Jack or Colby cheese

Sauté onion, bell pepper, and thyme in butter in medium
saucepan until tender, about 5 minutes. Stir in flour and cook
1 minute; add milk gradually. Heat to boiling over medium heat,
stirring constantly. Stir in crabmeat, avocados, and lemon juice.
Season to taste with salt and cayenne pepper. Spoon into lightly
greased 1-quart casserole; sprinkle with cheese. Broil for 2 minutes
or until golden.

Makes 6 servings.

Nutritional Analysis per Serving

Vitamin A	208.2 RE	Vitamin D	0.9 µg
Thiamin (B-1)	0.2 mg	Vitamin E	1.8 mg
Riboflavin (B-2)	0.3 mg	Calcium	259.9 mg
Niacin	2.5 mg	Iron	1.9 mg
Vitamin B-6	0.3 mg	Phosphorus	364.4 mg
Vitamin B-12	0.7 µg	Magnesium	71.1 mg
Folate (total)	85.9 µg	Zinc	4.3 mg
Vitamin C	26.1 mg	Potassium	832.5 mg

Savory Sole Casserole

PER SERVING: 133.0 CALORIES — 22.5 g PROTEIN — 2.9 g CARBOHYDRATE — 0.6 g FIBER —
3.1 g TOTAL FAT — 0.9 g SATURATED FAT — 59.3 mg CHOLESTEROL — 369.8 mg SODIUM

1 1/2 pounds skinless fillet of sole

1/2 cup (2 ounces) shredded reduced-fat Swiss cheese

1/4 cup finely chopped green onions

1 can (4 ounces) mushrooms, finely chopped

1/2 can (10 3/4 ounces) cream of shrimp soup (condensed)

1/2 teaspoon prepared mustard

1 teaspoon finely chopped parsley

Pinch ground nutmeg

Salt and cayenne pepper, to taste

Paprika, as garnish

Arrange fillets in single layer in shallow 6 x 10-inch baking dish; sprinkle with cheese and green onions. Combine remaining ingredients, except salt, cayenne pepper, and paprika, in small saucepan. Heat to boiling, stirring constantly; season to taste with salt and cayenne pepper. Pour over fish; sprinkle with paprika. Bake at 375 degrees, uncovered, 20 minutes, or until fish is tender and flakes with a fork.

Makes 6 servings.

Nutritional Analysis per Serving

Vitamin A	19.1 RE	Vitamin D	0.0 µg
Thiamin (B-1)	0.1 mg	Vitamin E	0.0 mg
Riboflavin (B-2)	0.1 mg	Calcium	112.4 mg
Niacin	2.0 mg	Iron	1.1 mg
Vitamin B-6	0 mg	Phosphorus	401.7 mg
Vitamin B-12	9.8 µg	Magnesium	37.3 mg
Folate (total)	15.4 µg	Zinc	1.0 mg
Vitamin C	1.1 mg	Potassium	410.3 mg

Kent's Seafood Casserole

PER SERVING: 405.1 CALORIES — 29.0 g PROTEIN — 23.4 g CARBOHYDRATE — 0.1 g FIBER —
20.5 g TOTAL FAT — 9.7 g SATURATED FAT — 105.6 mg CHOLESTEROL — 720.9 mg SODIUM

4 tablespoons butter or margarine

$^1/_4$ cup all-purpose flour

2 cups 2% milk

1 can (10$^3/_4$ ounces) reduced-sodium, reduced-fat cream of shrimp soup (condensed)

1 can (10$^3/_4$ ounces) reduced-sodium, reduced-fat
cream of mushroom soup (condensed)

$^1/_2$ cup shredded reduced-fat Cheddar cheese

1$^1/_2$ pounds fish fillets, baked and flaked

$^1/_2$ cup crushed cornflakes

Melt butter in medium saucepan over medium heat; add flour, stirring 1 to 2 minutes. Whisk in milk and heat to boiling; boil while whisking until thickened, 1 to 2 minutes. Stir in soups, cheese, and fish; cook, whisking, until cheese is melted, 2 to 3 minutes. Pour into 13 x 9-inch casserole and sprinkle with cornflakes. Bake, uncovered, at 350 degrees until hot through, about 20 minutes.

Makes 6 servings.

Nutritional Analysis per Serving

Vitamin A	359.4 RE	Vitamin D	1.0 µg
Thiamin (B-1)	0.3 mg	Vitamin E	0.2 mg
Riboflavin (B-2)	0.5 mg	Calcium	241.0 mg
Niacin	1.0 mg	Iron	1.8 mg
Vitamin B-6	0.2 mg	Phosphorus	452.7 mg
Vitamin B-12	0.4 µg	Magnesium	52.8 mg
Folate (total)	19.1 µg	Zinc	1.9 mg
Vitamin C	11.0 mg	Potassium	704.1 mg

Cheddar Cod

PER SERVING: 201.0 CALORIES — 26.2 g PROTEIN — 6.4 g CARBOHYDRATE — 0.1 g FIBER — 6.9 g TOTAL FAT — 4.1 g SATURATED FAT — 67.8 mg CHOLESTEROL — 258.5 mg SODIUM

1 pound skinless cod fillets
2 teaspoons lemon juice
1 tablespoon butter or margarine
2 tablespoons flour
1 cup fat-free milk
$^1/_2$ cup (2 ounces) shredded reduced-fat Cheddar cheese
$^1/_2$ teaspoon Dijon mustard
Salt and pepper, to taste

Place cod into a shallow baking dish; sprinkle with lemon juice. Combine butter, flour, and milk in small saucepan. Heat to boiling over medium heat, whisking constantly. Stir in cheese and mustard; season to taste with salt and pepper. Pour sauce over cod and bake, uncovered, at 350 degrees until fish is tender and flakes with a fork, about 20 minutes.

Makes 4 servings.

Nutritional Analysis per Serving

Vitamin A	122.9 RE	Vitamin D	1.9 µg
Thiamin (B-1)	0.1 mg	Vitamin E	0.3 mg
Riboflavin (B-2)	0.2 mg	Calcium	195.1 mg
Niacin	2.6 mg	Iron	0.6 mg
Vitamin B-6	0.3 mg	Phosphorus	372.3 mg
Vitamin B-12	1.3 µg	Magnesium	48.1 mg
Folate (total)	17.1 µg	Zinc	1.4 mg
Vitamin C	2.7 mg	Potassium	600.8 mg

Golden Shrimp Casserole

PER SERVING: 367.6 CALORIES — 33.9 g PROTEIN — 20.32 g CARBOHYDRATE — 1.2 g FIBER —
16.1 g TOTAL FAT — 7.8 g SATURATED FAT — 309.7 mg CHOLESTEROL — 1,048.8 mg SODIUM

8 slices white or wheat bread, crusts removed, cubed

2 cups (8 ounces) shredded sharp Cheddar cheese

1 1/2 pounds cooked shrimp, peeled, finely chopped

1 can (4 ounces) mushrooms, drained, finely chopped

4 eggs

2 3/4 cups fat-free milk, divided

1 teaspoon dry mustard

1/2 teaspoon salt

1/2 teaspoon pepper

1 can (10 3/4 ounces) cream of shrimp soup (condensed)

Place bread cubes into a lightly greased 9 x 13-inch baking
pan; sprinkle with cheese. Arrange shrimp and mushrooms over
cheese. Beat eggs, 2 1/4 cups milk, dry mustard, salt, and pepper in
medium bowl until well blended; pour over shrimp and mushroom mixture. Refrigerate, covered, overnight.

Blend cream of shrimp soup and remaining 1/2 cup milk; pour
over casserole. Bake at 350 degrees, uncovered, 1 hour, or until
puffed and golden brown.

Makes 8 servings.

Nutritional Analysis per Serving

Vitamin A	233.8 RE	Vitamin D	1.3 µg
Thiamin (B-1)	0.2 mg	Vitamin E	0.9 mg
Riboflavin (B-2)	0.5 mg	Calcium	387.3 mg
Niacin	3.4 mg	Iron	4.2 mg
Vitamin B-6	0.2 mg	Phosphorus	422.6 mg
Vitamin B-12	2.1 µg	Magnesium	54.8 mg
Folate (total)	48.2 µg	Zinc	3.0 mg
Vitamin C	2.7 mg	Potassium	419.2 mg

Shrimp and Mushroom Casserole

PER SERVING: 420.2 CALORIES — 29.1 g PROTEIN — 19.2 g CARBOHYDRATE — 0.5 g FIBER — 24.0 g TOTAL FAT — 4.6 g SATURATED FAT — 352.9 mg CHOLESTEROL — 1,119.4 mg SODIUM

1 pound cooked shrimp, peeled, finely chopped
1 can (10³/₄ ounces) reduced-sodium, reduced-fat cream of mushroom soup (condensed)
1 cup reduced-fat mayonnaise
¹/₄ cup finely chopped pimentos
1 clove of garlic, minced
2 teaspoons Worcestershire sauce
2 hard-cooked eggs, peeled, finely chopped
Salt and pepper, to taste
¹/₃ cup seasoned dry bread crumbs

Combine all ingredients, except salt, pepper, and bread crumbs, into large bowl, mixing well. Season to taste with salt and pepper. Spoon into lightly greased 3-quart casserole. Sprinkle with bread crumbs. Bake, uncovered, at 350 degrees until bubbly, about 20 minutes.

Makes 4 servings.

Nutritional Analysis per Serving

Vitamin A	190.8 RE	Vitamin D	0.3 µg
Thiamin (B-1)	0.1 mg	Vitamin E	3.3 mg
Riboflavin (B-2)	0.3 mg	Calcium	147.7 mg
Niacin	3.9 mg	Iron	4.8 mg
Vitamin B-6	0.2 mg	Phosphorus	248.4 mg
Vitamin B-12	2.1 µg	Magnesium	47.2 mg
Folate (total)	30.1 µg	Zinc	2.3 mg
Vitamin C	13.1 mg	Potassium	592.9 mg

Baked Shrimp and Cheese Puff

PER SERVING: 256.6 CALORIES — 24.6 g PROTEIN — 13.3 g CARBOHYDRATE — 0.4 g FIBER —
11.8 g TOTAL FAT — 6.4 g SATURATED FAT — 208.4 mg CHOLESTEROL — 762.1 mg SODIUM

4 slices bread, cut into 1/2-inch cubes
1/2 pound cooked shrimp, peeled, finely chopped
2 cups (8 ounces) shredded reduced-fat Monterey Jack or Colby cheese
3 eggs, lightly beaten
2 cups fat-free milk
1 teaspoon dry mustard
1/2 teaspoon salt
1/4 teaspoon cayenne pepper

Layer bread, shrimp, and cheese into lightly greased 11/2-quart casserole. Whisk remaining ingredients in small bowl; pour over casserole. Bake, uncovered, at 350 degrees until puffed and golden, 35 to 45 minutes.

Makes 6 servings.

Nutritional Analysis per Serving

Vitamin A	285.7 RE	Vitamin D	1.1 µg
Thiamin (B-1)	0.1 mg	Vitamin E	0.6 mg
Riboflavin (B-2)	0.5 mg	Calcium	413.1 mg
Niacin	1.7 mg	Iron	2.1 mg
Vitamin B-6	0.1 mg	Phosphorus	394.6 mg
Vitamin B-12	1.4 µg	Magnesium	39.1 mg
Folate (total)	33.3 µg	Zinc	3.3 mg
Vitamin C	1.7 mg	Potassium	318.6 mg

Lobster and Mushroom Casserole

PER SERVING: 288.6 CALORIES — 22.9 g PROTEIN — 20.9 g CARBOHYDRATE — 1.7 g FIBER —
12.8 g TOTAL FAT — 6.4 g SATURATED FAT — 191.6 mg CHOLESTEROL — 370.0 mg SODIUM

1 pound mushrooms, finely chopped

2 tablespoons butter or margarine

3 tablespoons flour

1 1/2 cups fat-free milk

1/2 cup reduced-sodium, fat-free chicken broth

2 cups lobster meat, finely chopped

Salt and pepper, to taste

2 egg yolks

1/2 cup reduced-fat sour cream

1/4 cup seasoned dry bread crumbs

Sauté mushrooms in butter in large skillet until tender, about
5 minutes. Stir in flour; cook 1 minute. Stir in milk and chicken
broth; heat to boiling over medium heat, stirring constantly. Stir in
lobster; season to taste with salt and pepper. Beat egg yolks and
sour cream in bowl and stir into lobster mixture. Pour into lightly
greased 9 x 13-inch casserole; sprinkle with bread crumbs. Bake,
uncovered, at 450 degrees until puffed and golden brown, about
10 minutes.

Makes 4 servings.

Nutritional Analysis per Serving

Vitamin A	231.8 RE	Vitamin D	3.5 µg
Thiamin (B-1)	0.3 mg	Vitamin E	1.4 mg
Riboflavin (B-2)	0.8 mg	Calcium	235.3 mg
Niacin	6.1 mg	Iron	2.4 mg
Vitamin B-6	0.2 mg	Phosphorus	366.4 mg
Vitamin B-12	1.1 µg	Magnesium	39.8 mg
Folate (total)	50.8 µg	Zinc	3.3 mg
Vitamin C	3.5 mg	Potassium	782.2 mg

Seafood Quiche

PER SERVING: 411.4 CALORIES — 21.3 g PROTEIN — 24.2 g CARBOHYDRATE — 0.9 g FIBER —
24.9 g TOTAL FAT — 6.1 g SATURATED FAT — 270.0 mg CHOLESTEROL — 567.4 mg SODIUM

3/4 cup flaked crabmeat
3/4 cup finely chopped cooked, peeled shrimp
1 cup (4 ounces) shredded reduced-fat Swiss cheese
1/3 cup finely chopped celery
1/3 cup finely chopped green onions
1 unbaked 9-inch pie crust
2/3 cup reduced-fat mayonnaise
1/4 cup all-purpose flour
1 cup fat-free milk
6 eggs

Combine crabmeat, shrimp, cheese, celery, and green onions
in large bowl. Spoon into pie crust. Whisk together mayonnaise,
flour, milk, and eggs in medium bowl; pour over seafood mixture
in pie crust. Bake at 375 degrees until browned and set, about
30 minutes.

Makes 6 servings.

Nutritional Analysis per Serving

Vitamin A	161.0 RE	Vitamin D	1.1 µg
Thiamin (B-1)	0.2 mg	Vitamin E	1.9 mg
Riboflavin (B-2)	0.5 mg	Calcium	280.2 mg
Niacin	2.3 mg	Iron	2.6 mg
Vitamin B-6	0.2 mg	Phosphorus	331.6 mg
Vitamin B-12	2.3 µg	Magnesium	33.2 mg
Folate (total)	69.4 µg	Zinc	2.5 mg
Vitamin C	2.8 mg	Potassium	292.9 mg

Seafood Casserole

PER SERVING: 365.3 CALORIES — 20.1 g PROTEIN — 25.2 g CARBOHYDRATE — 3.0 g FIBER — 20.0 g TOTAL FAT — 3.0 g SATURATED FAT — 110.0 mg CHOLESTEROL — 900.4 mg SODIUM

1 can (4 ounces) shrimp, drained, finely chopped
1 can (6¹/₂ ounces) crabmeat, drained, finely flaked
1 cup finely chopped celery
1 cup finely chopped onion
1 cup finely chopped green bell pepper
1 cup reduced-fat mayonnaise
Salt and pepper, to taste
1 tablespoon Worcestershire sauce
¹/₂ cup fat-free milk
1 cup herb-seasoned stuffing mix

Combine all ingredients in large bowl, mixing well. Pour into lightly greased 11 x 7-inch baking dish. Bake, uncovered, at 350 degrees until hot and bubbly, about 30 minutes.
Makes 4 servings.

Nutritional Analysis per Serving

Vitamin A	88.4 RE	Vitamin D	0.3 µg
Thiamin (B-1)	0.2 mg	Vitamin E	3.5 mg
Riboflavin (B-2)	0.2 mg	Calcium	143.9 mg
Niacin	2.5 mg	Iron	2.3 mg
Vitamin B-6	0.3 mg	Phosphorus	276.8 mg
Vitamin B-12	0.8 µg	Magnesium	45.1 mg
Folate (total)	49.4 µg	Zinc	2.6 mg
Vitamin C	40.3 mg	Potassium	535.8 mg

Ham with Sweet Potatoes

PER SERVING: 458.1 CALORIES — 18.1 g PROTEIN — 69.0 g CARBOHYDRATE — 3.3 g FIBER —
13.2 g TOTAL FAT — 6.0 g SATURATED FAT — 103.2 mg CHOLESTEROL — 1,053.9 mg SODIUM

2 cups twice-ground smoked ham
1 egg, lightly beaten
1/2 cup fat-free milk
1 1/2 cups fresh white bread crumbs
1 teaspoon dry mustard, divided
1 can (16 ounces) sweet potatoes, drained
2 tablespoons melted butter or margarine
1/2 cup honey
2 tablespoons cider vinegar

Combine ham, egg, milk, bread crumbs, and 1/2 teaspoon of
the mustard in medium bowl. Mix until well blended, then shape
into 12 meatballs. Place in lightly greased 13 x 9-inch baking
dish. Arrange sweet potatoes between meatballs in dish. Combine
melted butter, honey, vinegar, and remaining 1/2 teaspoon mustard;
drizzle over ham and potatoes. Bake, uncovered, at 375 degrees
until lightly browned and bubbly, about 40 minutes.

Makes 4 servings.

Nutritional Analysis per Serving

Vitamin A	747.8 RE	Vitamin D	0.6 µg
Thiamin (B-1)	0.5 mg	Vitamin E	0.7 mg
Riboflavin (B-2)	0.4 mg	Calcium	89.5 mg
Niacin	4.5 mg	Iron	2.6 mg
Vitamin B-6	0.3 mg	Phosphorus	253.7 mg
Vitamin B-12	0.6 µg	Magnesium	37.7 mg
Folate (total)	34.1 µg	Zinc	2.1 mg
Vitamin C	12.4 mg	Potassium	549.7 mg

Cheesy Ham and Potato Bake

PER SERVING: 253.9 CALORIES — 14.7 g PROTEIN — 31.5 g CARBOHYDRATE — 2.6 g FIBER —
7.2 g TOTAL FAT — 3.7 g SATURATED FAT — 34.3 mg CHOLESTEROL — 910.4 mg SODIUM

1 1/2 cups finely chopped ham
1 can (10 3/4 ounces) low-sodium, reduced-fat cream of mushroom soup (condensed)
1/4 cup fat-free milk
1 tablespoon instant minced onion
1/8 teaspoon pepper
1 cup (4 ounces) shredded reduced-fat sharp Cheddar cheese, divided
4 cups cooked finely diced potatoes
1 cup finely shredded carrots
3/4 cup fresh white or wheat bread crumbs

Combine ham, mushroom soup, milk, minced onion, pepper, and 1/2 cup cheese, mixing well. Arrange potatoes in lightly greased 2-quart baking dish; top with carrots, then top with ham mixture. Mix bread crumbs and remaining 1/2 cup cheese and sprinkle over casserole. Bake, uncovered, at 350 degrees until lightly browned and bubbly, about 45 minutes.

Makes 6 servings.

Nutritional Analysis per Serving

Vitamin A	582.0 RE	Vitamin D	0.1 µg
Thiamin (B-1)	0.5 mg	Vitamin E	0.3 mg
Riboflavin (B-2)	0.2 mg	Calcium	212.3 mg
Niacin	3.6 mg	Iron	0.9 mg
Vitamin B-6	0.5 mg	Phosphorus	243.9 mg
Vitamin B-12	0.5 µg	Magnesium	38.1 mg
Folate (total)	20.5 µg	Zinc	1.9 mg
Vitamin C	10.1 mg	Potassium	775.0 mg

Deviled Ham

PER SERVING: 107.9 CALORIES — 13.5 g PROTEIN — 1.7 g CARBOHYDRATE — 0.0 g FIBER —
4.6 g TOTAL FAT — 2.9 g SATURATED FAT — 36.2 mg CHOLESTEROL — 1,185.7 mg SODIUM

2 cups diced smoked ham
2 tablespoons reduced-fat mayonnaise
1¹/₂ tablespoons Dijon mustard
¹/₄ teaspoon hot pepper sauce

Process all ingredients in food processor until very finely chopped.

Makes 3 servings.

Serve on soft bread or over a baked potato**

**Nutritional information does not include the bread or potato accompaniment

Nutritional Analysis per Serving

Vitamin A	0.7 RE	Vitamin D	0.0 µg
Thiamin (B-1)	0.0 mg	Vitamin E	0.7 mg
Riboflavin (B-2)	0.0 mg	Calcium	0.1 mg
Niacin	0.0 mg	Iron	0.6 mg
Vitamin B-6	0.0 mg	Phosphorus	0.1 mg
Vitamin B-12	0.0 µg	Magnesium	0.1 mg
Folate (total)	0.0 µg	Zinc	0.0 mg
Vitamin C	0.0 mg	Potassium	1.6 mg

Beef and Broccoli Casserole

PER SERVING: 416.0 CALORIES — 27.7 g PROTEIN — 28.4 g CARBOHYDRATE — 4.4 g FIBER — 20.6 g TOTAL FAT — 10.0 g SATURATED FAT — 126.8 mg CHOLESTEROL — 861.9 mg SODIUM

$1/2$ pound twice-ground lean beef
3 cups finely chopped cooked broccoli
$1/2$ cup evaporated milk
1 egg, lightly beaten
1 can ($10^3/4$ ounces) reduced-sodium, reduced-fat
cream of chicken soup (condensed)
1 cup (4 ounces) shredded reduced-fat Cheddar cheese
1 cup herb stuffing mix

Cook beef in large skillet over medium-high heat until browned, about 5 minutes, crumbling finely with fork; drain fat. Stir in broccoli, milk, egg, and chicken soup. Pour into a lightly greased $1^1/2$-quart casserole. Combine cheese and stuffing mix; sprinkle over casserole. Bake, uncovered, at 350 degrees for 25 minutes, or until lightly browned.

NOTE: Cooked asparagus, cauliflower, eggplant, or zucchini can be substituted for the broccoli.

Makes 4 servings.

Nutritional Analysis per Serving

Vitamin A	357.0 RE	Vitamin D	0.8 µg
Thiamin (B-1)	0.2 mg	Vitamin E	2.2 mg
Riboflavin (B-2)	0.6 mg	Calcium	359.5 mg
Niacin	4.0 mg	Iron	2.9 mg
Vitamin B-6	0.3 mg	Phosphorus	385.2 mg
Vitamin B-12	1.3 µg	Magnesium	56.2 mg
Folate (total)	70.1 µg	Zinc	4.4 mg
Vitamin C	103.1 mg	Potassium	658.2 mg

Beef, Vegetable, and Egg Scramble

PER SERVING: 363.7 CALORIES — 27.2 g PROTEIN — 7.7 g CARBOHYDRATE — 2.7 g FIBER —
24.6 g TOTAL FAT — 9.3 g SATURATED FAT — 223.9 mg CHOLESTEROL — 158.1 mg SODIUM

1 1/2 pounds twice-ground lean beef

2 small onions, finely chopped

2 cloves garlic, minced

1/2 pound mushrooms, finely chopped

1 teaspoon dried oregano leaves

1/2 teaspoon pepper

1/4 teaspoon ground nutmeg

1 package (10 ounces) frozen chopped spinach, thawed, well drained

4 eggs, lightly beaten

Salt, to taste

Cook ground beef in large skillet over medium-high heat until browned, about 5 minutes, crumbling finely with a fork. Add onions, garlic, and mushrooms; cook over medium heat, stirring occasionally, until onions are soft, about 5 minutes. Stir in oregano, pepper, nutmeg, and spinach; cook about 3 minutes longer. Add eggs; stir mixture over low heat just until eggs begin to set, about 2 minutes. Season to taste with salt.

Makes 6 servings.

Nutritional Analysis per Serving

Vitamin A	432.1 RE	Vitamin D	1.2 µg
Thiamin (B-1)	0.1 mg	Vitamin E	1.1 mg
Riboflavin (B-2)	0.7 mg	Calcium	93.8 mg
Niacin	6.4 mg	Iron	4.1 mg
Vitamin B-6	0.4 mg	Phosphorus	286.9 mg
Vitamin B-12	2.3 µg	Magnesium	60.0 mg
Folate (total)	91.0 µg	Zinc	5.3 mg
Vitamin C	15.2 mg	Potassium	697.1 mg

Cheesy Meat Loaf

PER SERVING: 389.2 CALORIES — 33.7 g PROTEIN — 13.6 g CARBOHYDRATE — 1.4 g FIBER —
21.9 g TOTAL FAT — 8.7 g SATURATED FAT — 135.7 mg CHOLESTEROL — 924.2 mg SODIUM

1 pound twice-ground lean beef
1 cup 1% low-fat cottage cheese
1 egg
$1/2$ cup quick-cooking oats
$1/4$ cup catsup
1 tablespoon prepared mustard
2 tablespoons finely chopped onion
$1/2$ teaspoon salt
$1/4$ teaspoon pepper
$1/4$ cup (1 ounce) grated Parmesan cheese

Combine all ingredients, except Parmesan cheese, in large
bowl. Mix until well blended. Form into loaf in 11 x 7-inch
baking pan. Bake, uncovered, at 350 degrees until juices run clear
and meat thermometer registers 170 degrees, about 45 minutes.
Sprinkle with Parmesan cheese during last 10 minutes of baking
time. Let stand 5 minutes before serving.

Makes 4 servings.

Nutritional Analysis per Serving

Vitamin A	54.6 RE	Vitamin D	0.2 µg
Thiamin (B-1)	0.1 mg	Vitamin E	0.8 mg
Riboflavin (B-2)	0.5 mg	Calcium	129.7 mg
Niacin	5.0 mg	Iron	3.2 mg
Vitamin B-6	0.3 mg	Phosphorus	355.0 mg
Vitamin B-12	2.3 µg	Magnesium	61.8 mg
Folate (total)	27.8 µg	Zinc	5.6 mg
Vitamin C	2.7 mg	Potassium	514.3 mg

Barbecue Meat Loaf

PER SERVING: 255.3 CALORIES — 18.8 g PROTEIN — 8.7 g CARBOHYDRATE — 0.6 g FIBER —
15.5 g TOTAL FAT — 5.9 g SATURATED FAT — 111.3 mg CHOLESTEROL — 765.6 mg SODIUM

2 cups fresh white bread crumbs

1/2 cup finely chopped onion

1 tablespoon prepared horseradish

2 teaspoons celery salt

2 teaspoons liquid smoke

1 teaspoon garlic salt

1/4 teaspoon pepper

2 eggs

1 1/2 pounds twice-ground lean beef

1/2 cup barbecue sauce

Combine all ingredients, except barbecue sauce, in large bowl;
mix well. Press lightly into 5 x 9-inch ungreased loaf pan, or
form into loaf in 7 x 11-inch baking pan; bake, uncovered, at
350 degrees, about 30 minutes. Pour off any fat that has accumu-
lated in pan. Spoon barbecue sauce over meatloaf and continue
baking until juices run clear and meat thermometer registers
170 degrees, about 30 minutes.

Makes 8 servings.

Nutritional Analysis per Serving

Vitamin A	40.8 RE	Vitamin D	0.2 µg
Thiamin (B-1)	0.1 mg	Vitamin E	0.5 mg
Riboflavin (B-2)	0.3 mg	Calcium	31.5 mg
Niacin	4.1 mg	Iron	2.4 mg
Vitamin B-6	0.2 mg	Phosphorus	160.7 mg
Vitamin B-12	1.4 µg	Magnesium	25.1 mg
Folate (total)	24.1 µg	Zinc	3.8 mg
Vitamin C	1.8 mg	Potassium	319.6 mg

Hamburger-Green Bean Casserole

PER SERVING: 315.4 CALORIES — 21.9 g PROTEIN — 19.8 g CARBOHYDRATE — 5.1 g FIBER —
17.2 g TOTAL FAT — 6.2 g SATURATED FAT — 57.8 mg CHOLESTEROL — 926.3 mg SODIUM

1 pound twice-ground lean beef
1 medium onion, finely chopped
1 can (10^3/$_4$ ounces) tomato soup (condensed)
^{1}/$_4$ teaspoon pepper
1 can (15 ounces) green beans, drained
3 cups mashed potatoes
4 slices (3 ounces) reduced-fat American cheese

Cook hamburger and onion in large skillet over medium-high heat until beef is browned, about 5 minutes, crumbling finely with a fork. Stir in tomato soup and pepper; spoon mixture into lightly greased 2-quart casserole. Place green beans on top; spread potatoes over beans. Top with cheese. Bake, uncovered, at 350 degrees until lightly browned, about 30 minutes.

Makes 6 servings.

Nutritional Analysis per Serving

Vitamin A	148.2 RE	Vitamin D	0.5 µg
Thiamin (B-1)	0.1 mg	Vitamin E	2.7 mg
Riboflavin (B-2)	0.3 mg	Calcium	162.9 mg
Niacin	5.0 mg	Iron	3.5 mg
Vitamin B-6	0.3 mg	Phosphorus	256.6 mg
Vitamin B-12	1.4 µg	Magnesium	50.8 mg
Folate (total)	50.3 µg	Zinc	4.1 mg
Vitamin C	17.1 mg	Potassium	792.6 mg

Hamburger Stew

PER SERVING: 311.4 CALORIES — 17.9 g PROTEIN — 35.0 g CARBOHYDRATE —7.0 g FIBER —
12.0 g TOTAL FAT — 4.5 g SATURATED FAT — 46.6 mg CHOLESTEROL — 1,150.0 mg SODIUM

1 pound twice-ground lean beef
1 teaspoon garlic salt
1 cup finely shredded cabbage
1 cup cooked carrots, shredded
1 cup cooked potatoes, shredded
2 cups barbecue sauce
2 cans (15 ounces each) pork and beans

Brown beef and garlic salt in skillet. In large saucepan, cook cabbage in 2 cups water until tender. Add beef and remaining ingredients. Bring to a boil. Reduce heat. Let simmer for 30 minutes.

Makes 8 servings.

Nutritional Analysis per Serving

Vitamin A	547.0 RE	Vitamin D	0.0 µg
Thiamin (B-1)	0.1 mg	Vitamin E	1.5 mg
Riboflavin (B-2)	0.2 mg	Calcium	87.1 mg
Niacin	4.0 mg	Iron	5.4 mg
Vitamin B-6	0.4 mg	Phosphorus	232.5 mg
Vitamin B-12	1.2 µg	Magnesium	67.5 mg
Folate (total)	39.7 µg	Zinc	8.8 mg
Vitamin C	12.4 mg	Potassium	718.1 mg

Spinach and Beef Frittata

PER SERVING: 362.6 CALORIES — 31.0 g PROTEIN — 8.1 g CARBOHYDRATE — 3.3 g FIBER — 22.9 g TOTAL FAT — 8.5 g SATURATED FAT — 289.1 mg CHOLESTEROL — 225.1 mg SODIUM

1 1/2 pounds twice-ground lean beef

1 small onion, minced

2 packages (10 ounces each) frozen chopped spinach, thawed, well drained

1 teaspoon minced garlic

1 teaspoon dried oregano leaves

Salt and pepper, to taste

6 eggs

1/4 cup fat-free milk

Cook ground beef and onion in skillet until beef is browned, about 5 minutes, crumbling beef finely with a fork. Stir in spinach, garlic, and oregano; season to taste with salt and pepper. Beat eggs and milk until blended; stir into spinach mixture and cook over low heat until eggs are cooked, stirring occasionally.

Makes 6 servings.

Nutritional Analysis per Serving

Vitamin A	838.6 RE	Vitamin D	0.8 µg
Thiamin (B-1)	0.1 mg	Vitamin E	1.6 mg
Riboflavin (B-2)	0.7 mg	Calcium	191.4 mg
Niacin	5.1 mg	Iron	4.5 mg
Vitamin B-6	0.4 mg	Phosphorus	311.8 mg
Vitamin B-12	2.3 µg	Magnesium	96.6 mg
Folate (total)	136.6 µg	Zinc	6.0 mg
Vitamin C	13.2 mg	Potassium	716.0 mg

Beef–Cabbage Casserole

PER SERVING: 447.7 CALORIES — 30.0 g PROTEIN — 31.3 g CARBOHYDRATE — 7.0 g FIBER —
23.0 g TOTAL FAT — 10.0 g SATURATED FAT — 91.2 mg CHOLESTEROL — 958.4 mg SODIUM

1 small head cabbage, finely chopped
1 pound twice-ground lean beef
$1/2$ cup minced onion
$1/2$ cup cooked rice
$1/2$ teaspoon salt
$1/4$ teaspoon pepper
1 can ($10^3/4$ ounces) tomato soup (condensed)
$1^1/2$ cups water
$1/2$ cup (2 ounces) shredded Cheddar cheese

Sprinkle cabbage over the bottom of a 9 x 13-inch baking dish. Cook ground beef and onion in large skillet until meat is browned, about 8 minutes, crumbling finely with a fork. Stir in rice, salt, and pepper and mix well. Spoon beef mixture over cabbage.

Mix tomato soup and water in small saucepan; heat to boiling. Pour over beef and cabbage mixture. Bake, covered, at 350 degrees, about 1 hour. Uncover, sprinkle with cheese, and bake until cheese is melted, about 5 minutes. Stir lightly before serving.

Makes 4 servings.

NOTE: For a spicier flavor, use 1 can (8 ounces) herb-seasoned tomato sauce in place of tomato soup.

Nutritional Analysis per Serving

Vitamin A	100.5 RE	Vitamin D	0.0 µg
Thiamin (B-1)	0.2 mg	Vitamin E	0.5 mg
Riboflavin (B-2)	0.4 mg	Calcium	235.9 mg
Niacin	6.1 mg	Iron	4.4 mg
Vitamin B-6	0.4 mg	Phosphorus	299.7 mg
Vitamin B-12	1.9 µg	Magnesium	65.3 mg
Folate (total)	121.8 µg	Zinc	5.7 mg
Vitamin C	75.9 mg	Potassium	934.3 mg

Baked Chili

PER SERVING: 369.7 CALORIES — 26.9 g PROTEIN — 16.7 g CARBOHYDRATE — 3.0 g FIBER — 21.2 g TOTAL FAT — 9.0 g SATURATED FAT — 86.3 mg CHOLESTEROL — 692.5 mg SODIUM

1 pound twice-ground lean beef

$^1/_2$ cup finely chopped celery

1 medium onion, finely chopped

1 can (10$^3/_4$ ounces) tomato soup (condensed)

$^3/_4$ cup water

1 tablespoon paprika

1–2 tablespoons chili powder

$^1/_4$–$^1/_2$ teaspoon garlic powder

$^1/_8$ teaspoon ground allspice

Salt and pepper, to taste

$^1/_2$ cup (2 ounces) shredded reduced-fat sharp Cheddar cheese

Cook ground beef, celery, and onion in large skillet until beef is browned, about 8 minutes, crumbling finely with a fork. Mix in tomato soup, water, paprika, chili powder, garlic powder, and allspice. Season to taste with salt and pepper.

Transfer mixture to 1$^1/_2$-quart casserole. Bake, covered, at 350 degrees until hot through, 30 to 45 minutes. Sprinkle cheese over top, and bake, uncovered, until cheese melts, about 5 minutes.

Makes 4 servings.

Nutritional Analysis per Serving

Vitamin A	242.3 RE	Vitamin D	0.0 µg
Thiamin (B-1)	0.1 mg	Vitamin E	0.3 mg
Riboflavin (B-2)	0.4 mg	Calcium	140.9 mg
Niacin	5.6 mg	Iron	3.4 mg
Vitamin B-6	0.3 mg	Phosphorus	259.9 mg
Vitamin B-12	1.9 µg	Magnesium	37.5 mg
Folate (total)	19.4 µg	Zinc	5.5 mg
Vitamin C	6.8 mg	Potassium	507.6 mg

Country Pie

PER SERVING: 339.6 CALORIES — 22.3 g PROTEIN — 20.0 g CARBOHYDRATE — 1.9 g FIBER —
18.8 g TOTAL FAT — 8.7 g SATURATED FAT — 70.7 mg CHOLESTEROL — 752.4 mg SODIUM

1 pound twice-ground lean beef
2$^1/_2$ cups canned, reduced-sodium tomato sauce, divided
$^1/_2$ cup Italian-style dry bread crumbs
1 teaspoon salt
$^1/_8$ teaspoon pepper
1$^1/_3$ cups cooked rice
1 cup water
1 cup (4 ounces) shredded Cheddar cheese, divided
$^3/_4$ teaspoon dried Italian seasoning

Combine ground beef, 1 cup tomato sauce, bread crumbs, salt, and pepper in bowl; mix well. Press mixture onto bottom and against sides of 9-inch pie plate.

Mix rice, water, remaining 1$^1/_2$ cups tomato sauce, $^1/_2$ cup cheese, and Italian seasoning in saucepan; heat to boiling. Pour mixture into beef-lined pie plate. Cover and bake at 350 degrees until beef is cooked, about 30 minutes. Sprinkle with remaining $^1/_2$ cup cheese and bake, uncovered, until melted, about 5 minutes.

Makes 6 servings.

Nutritional Analysis per Serving

Vitamin A	110.0 RE	Vitamin D	0.1 µg
Thiamin (B-1)	0.1 mg	Vitamin E	0.2 mg
Riboflavin (B-2)	0.3 mg	Calcium	190.4 mg
Niacin	3.6 mg	Iron	3.3 mg
Vitamin B-6	0.1 mg	Phosphorus	218.2 mg
Vitamin B-12	1.3 µg	Magnesium	24.7 mg
Folate (total)	28.0 µg	Zinc	3.9 mg
Vitamin C	11.8 mg	Potassium	251.1 mg

Hot Tamale Casserole

PER SERVING: 354.5 CALORIES — 24.4 g PROTEIN — 22.6 g CARBOHYDRATE — 4.3 g FIBER —
19.0 g TOTAL FAT — 7.1 g SATURATED FAT — 76.3 mg CHOLESTEROL — 578.1 mg SODIUM

1 1/2 pounds twice-ground lean beef
2 medium onions, finely chopped
1 can (16 ounces) tomato sauce
3 tablespoons chili powder
1 teaspoon dried oregano leaves
Salt and pepper, to taste
1 1/2 cups water
3/4 cup yellow cornmeal

Cook ground beef and onions in large skillet over medium heat until beef is browned and onions are tender, about 10 minutes, crumbling beef finely with a fork; drain. Add tomato sauce, chili powder, and oregano and cook until thickened, about 5 minutes. Season to taste with salt and pepper.

Heat 1 1/2 cups of water to boiling in large saucepan; slowly stir in cornmeal. Reduce heat and simmer slowly, stirring constantly, until thick, 5 to 8 minutes; season to taste with salt. Pour cornmeal mixture into 2-quart casserole; top with beef mixture. Bake, covered, at 375 degrees for 20 minutes.

Makes 6 servings.

Nutritional Analysis per Serving

Vitamin A	219.2 RE	Vitamin D	0.0 µg
Thiamin (B-1)	0.2 mg	Vitamin E	1.4 mg
Riboflavin (B-2)	0.4 mg	Calcium	41.6 mg
Niacin	6.4 mg	Iron	4.1 mg
Vitamin B-6	0.4 mg	Phosphorus	245.3 mg
Vitamin B-12	1.8 µg	Magnesium	67.4 mg
Folate (total)	28.5 µg	Zinc	5.3 mg
Vitamin C	14.9 mg	Potassium	782.8 mg

Savory Beef Casserole

PER SERVING: 437.3 CALORIES — 26.0 g PROTEIN — 26.4 g CARBOHYDRATE — 2.5 g FIBER —
24.6 g TOTAL FAT — 10.0 g SATURATED FAT — 95.4 mg CHOLESTEROL — 1,159.6 mg SODIUM

2 pounds twice-ground lean beef

1–2 teaspoons salt

$^{1}/_{2}$ teaspoon pepper

1 large onion, finely chopped

$^{3}/_{4}$ teaspoon dried oregano leaves

$^{3}/_{4}$ teaspoon dried sage leaves

2–4 tablespoons butter or margarine

4 cups fresh whole wheat bread crumbs

$^{1}/_{3}$–$^{1}/_{2}$ cup reduced-sodium, reduced-fat chicken broth

2 cans (10$^{3}/_{4}$ ounces each) reduced-sodium,
reduced-fat cream of chicken soup (condensed)

2 cans (10$^{3}/_{4}$ ounces each) reduced-sodium,
reduced-fat cream of celery soup (condensed)

Paprika, as garnish

Mix ground beef, salt, and pepper; press into bottom of a
9 x 13-inch baking dish. Sauté onion, oregano, and sage in butter
in medium skillet until onion is tender, about 5 minutes. Toss
bread crumbs with onions and chicken broth; spoon evenly
over beef.

Mix the soups and pour over the bread crumb mixture.
Lightly sprinkle the top with paprika. Bake, uncovered, at
350 degrees until browned, about 45 minutes.

Makes 8 servings.

Nutritional Analysis per Serving

Vitamin A	94.5 RE	Vitamin D	0.1 µg
Thiamin (B-1)	0.1 mg	Vitamin E	0.6 mg
Riboflavin (B-2)	0.3 mg	Calcium	121.9 mg
Niacin	5.7 mg	Iron	2.9 mg
Vitamin B-6	0.2 mg	Phosphorus	212.3 mg
Vitamin B-12	1.8 µg	Magnesium	45.8 mg
Folate (total)	16.8 µg	Zinc	5.1 mg
Vitamin C	16.3 mg	Potassium	429.4 mg

Spaghetti Skillet Casserole

PER SERVING: 700.0 CALORIES — 41.5 g PROTEIN — 64.6 g CARBOHYDRATE — 2.8 g FIBER —
29.3 g TOTAL FAT — 13.2 g SATURATED FAT — 104.3 mg CHOLESTEROL — 1,183.6 mg SODIUM

1 pound twice-ground lean beef
1 onion, finely chopped
$1/2$ medium green bell pepper, finely chopped
1 can ($10^3/4$ ounces) reduced-sodium tomato soup (condensed)
1 can ($10^3/4$ ounces) reduced-sodium,
reduced-fat cream of mushroom soup (condensed)
1 cup water
$1^1/2$ cups (6 ounces) shredded reduced-fat Parmesan cheese, divided
8 ounces spaghetti, cooked, drained, and finely chopped
Salt and pepper, to taste

Cook ground beef, onion, and bell pepper in large skillet until
beef is browned and vegetables are tender, crumbling beef finely
with a fork. Stir in soups and 1 cup water and heat to boiling;
reduce heat and simmer, uncovered, for several minutes. Stir in
1 cup cheese and spaghetti; season to taste with salt and pepper.

Spoon mixture into $2^1/2$-quart casserole and sprinkle with
remaining $1/2$ cup cheese. Bake, uncovered, at 350 degrees until
bubbly, about 30 minutes.

Makes 4 servings.

Nutritional Analysis per Serving

Vitamin A	86.7 RE	Vitamin D	0.0 µg
Thiamin (B-1)	0.5 mg	Vitamin E	0.4 mg
Riboflavin (B-2)	0.6 mg	Calcium	463.9 mg
Niacin	8.4 mg	Iron	4.5 mg
Vitamin B-6	0.3 mg	Phosphorus	464.7 mg
Vitamin B-12	2.2 µg	Magnesium	65.4 mg
Folate (total)	109.1 µg	Zinc	6.4 mg
Vitamin C	30.3 mg	Potassium	867.3 mg

Colorado Hash

PER SERVING: 233.6 CALORIES — 13.1 g PROTEIN — 16.9 g CARBOHYDRATE — 2.3 g FIBER —
12.7 g TOTAL FAT — 3.7 g SATURATED FAT — 38.2 mg CHOLESTEROL — 202.8 mg SODIUM

3 medium onions, finely chopped

1 large green bell pepper, finely chopped

2–3 tablespoons canola oil

1 pound twice-ground lean beef

1 can (16 ounces) reduced-sodium herbed tomato sauce

$1/2$ cup uncooked rice

2–3 teaspoons chili powder

$1/2$ teaspoon dried thyme leaves

$1/2$–1 teaspoon salt

$1/4$ teaspoon pepper

Sauté onions and bell pepper in oil in large skillet until onions are golden-colored, 5 to 8 minutes.

Add ground beef and cook until browned, crumbling beef finely with a fork. Add remaining ingredients.

Spoon mixture into a 2-quart baking dish. Bake, covered, at 350 degrees for 30 minutes; remove cover and bake for an additional 15 minutes.

Makes 8 servings.

Nutritional Analysis per Serving

Vitamin A	64.1 RE	Vitamin D	0.0 µg
Thiamin (B-1)	0.1 mg	Vitamin E	1.0 mg
Riboflavin (B-2)	0.2 mg	Calcium	37.2 mg
Niacin	3.0 mg	Iron	2.4 mg
Vitamin B-6	0.2 mg	Phosphorus	111.3 mg
Vitamin B-12	0.9 µg	Magnesium	21.3 mg
Folate (total)	33.9 µg	Zinc	2.6 mg
Vitamin C	22.9 mg	Potassium	278.8 mg

Layered Casserole Italiano

PER SERVING: 308.3 CALORIES — 23.6 g PROTEIN — 21.8 g CARBOHYDRATE — 2.0 g FIBER —
14.3 g TOTAL FAT — 6.7 g SATURATED FAT — 55.4 mg CHOLESTEROL — 940.7 mg SODIUM

5 cups finely chopped zucchini

$1/2$ cup finely chopped onion

1 small clove garlic, minced

2 tablespoons butter or margarine

1 pound twice-ground lean beef

1 cup uncooked quick-cooking rice

1 teaspoon dried basil leaves

$3/4$ teaspoon salt

$1/2$ teaspoon pepper

1 carton (16 ounces) 1% cream-style cottage cheese

1 can ($10^3/4$ ounces) tomato soup (condensed)

$2/3$ cup water

1 cup (4 ounces) shredded reduced-fat sharp American cheese

Sauté zucchini, onion, and garlic in butter in large skillet until
tender, 5 to 8 minutes; add ground beef and cook until beef is
browned, crumbling finely with a fork. Stir in the rice, basil, salt,
and pepper.

Spoon the beef mixture into the bottom of a 2½-quart casserole; mix cottage cheese, tomato soup, and water; pour over the
top of casserole and sprinkle with cheese.

Bake, uncovered, at 350 degrees until hot and lightly
browned, about 40 minutes.

Makes 8 servings.

Nutritional Analysis per Serving

Vitamin A	136.8 RE	Vitamin D	0.1 µg
Thiamin (B-1)	0.2 mg	Vitamin E	0.3 mg
Riboflavin (B-2)	0.3 mg	Calcium	166.9 mg
Niacin	3.6 mg	Iron	2.4 mg
Vitamin B-6	0.2 mg	Phosphorus	259.9 mg
Vitamin B-12	0.4 µg	Magnesium	33.3 mg
Folate (total)	55.5 µg	Zinc	3.3 mg
Vitamin C	8.0 mg	Potassium	446.7 mg

Mexican Chili Casserole

PER SERVING: 444.3 CALORIES — 28.0 g PROTEIN — 25.8 g CARBOHYDRATE — 1.1 g FIBER —
24.6 g TOTAL FAT — 10.9 g SATURATED FAT — 71.8 mg CHOLESTEROL — 790.3 mg SODIUM

1 pound twice-ground lean beef
1 teaspoon dried oregano leaves
Salt and pepper, to taste
2 cups (8 ounces) shredded reduced-fat mozzarella cheese, divided
1 can (21 ounces) hot chili without beans
8 ounces finely crushed baked tortilla chips

Cook ground beef in large skillet until browned, crumbling
finely with a fork; add oregano and season to taste with salt and
pepper. Layer beef, 1 cup cheese, and the chili into a 1½-quart
casserole. Combine remaining 1 cup cheese and tortilla chips;
sprinkle over top of casserole. Bake, uncovered, at 375 degrees
until hot through and browned, about 30 minutes.

Makes 8 servings.

Nutritional Analysis per Serving

Vitamin A	102.6 RE	Vitamin D	.0 µg
Thiamin (B-1)	.0 mg	Vitamin E	0.1 mg
Riboflavin (B-2)	0.3 mg	Calcium	259.9 mg
Niacin	4.0 mg	Iron	2.6 mg
Vitamin B-6	0.1 mg	Phosphorus	343.6 mg
Vitamin B-12	1.2 µg	Magnesium	17.9 mg
Folate (total)	9.6 µg	Zinc	4.5 mg
Vitamin C	0.1 mg	Potassium	356.3 mg

Baked Chilies Rellenos

PER SERVING: 338.3 CALORIES — 29.1 g PROTEIN — 10.4 g CARBOHYDRATE — 1.7 g FIBER —
19.8 g TOTAL FAT — 8.7 g SATURATED FAT — 203.8 mg CHOLESTEROL — 850.5 mg SODIUM

1 pound twice-ground lean beef

1/2 cup finely chopped onion

1 teaspoon salt, divided

1/2 teaspoon black pepper, divided

2 cans (4 ounces each) hot or mild green chilies, finely chopped, divided

1 1/2 cups (6 ounces) shredded reduced-fat Cheddar cheese

4 eggs, beaten

1 1/2 cups fat-free milk

1/4 cup all-purpose flour

4 dashes hot pepper sauce

Cook ground beef and onion in large skillet until beef is
browned, crumbling beef finely with a fork; drain; stir in half the
salt and pepper.

Spoon 1 can green chilies into a 10 x 6-inch baking dish;
sprinkle with cheese and top with meat mixture. Spoon second
can of green chilies over the meat mixture.

Beat eggs, milk, flour, hot pepper sauce, and remaining salt
and pepper in bowl until smooth. Pour over mixture in baking
dish. Bake, uncovered, at 350 degrees until topping is set and
sharp knife inserted comes out clean, about 45 minutes. Let stand
5 minutes. Cut into squares to serve.

Makes 6 servings.

Nutritional Analysis per Serving

Vitamin A	221.1 RE	Vitamin D	1.1 µg
Thiamin (B-1)	0.1 mg	Vitamin E	0.5 mg
Riboflavin (B-2)	0.5 mg	Calcium	401.8 mg
Niacin	3.5 mg	Iron	2.3 mg
Vitamin B-6	0.2 mg	Phosphorus	238.1 mg
Vitamin B-12	1.7 µg	Magnesium	28.0 mg
Folate (total)	33.5 µg	Zinc	3.8 mg
Vitamin C	9.1 mg	Potassium	385.5 mg

Tuna–Vegetable Baked Potatoes

PER SERVING: 350.0 CALORIES — 18.7 g PROTEIN — 59.4 g CARBOHYDRATE — 5.6 g FIBER —
4.4 g TOTAL FAT — 2.5 g SATURATED FAT — 24.7 mg CHOLESTEROL — 233.5 mg SODIUM

2 tablespoons finely chopped onion

3 tablespoons finely chopped green bell pepper

1 tablespoon butter or margarine

1$^1/_2$ tablespoons flour

$^1/_4$ teaspoon onion powder

$^1/_4$ teaspoon garlic powder

$^1/_8$ teaspoon dried thyme leaves

$^1/_8$ teaspoon dried marjoram leaves

1 cup fat-free milk

2 tablespoons reduced-fat sour cream

$^1/_2$ cup thinly sliced carrots, cooked, drained

1 can (6 ounces) water-packed tuna, drained

Salt and pepper, to taste

4 medium Idaho potatoes, baked, warm

Sauté onion and bell pepper in butter until tender, about
3 minutes. Stir in flour, onion powder, garlic powder, thyme, and
marjoram. Cook 1 minute, stirring constantly; stir in milk. Heat
to boiling, stirring constantly. Stir in sour cream, carrots, and
tuna. Stir over medium heat until hot; season to taste with salt
and pepper. Serve over split baked potatoes.

Makes 4 servings.

Nutritional Analysis per Serving

Vitamin A	519.4 RE	Vitamin D	0.7 µg
Thiamin (B-1)	0.3 mg	Vitamin E	0.5 mg
Riboflavin (B-2)	0.2 mg	Calcium	124.1 mg
Niacin	9.4 mg	Iron	3.8 mg
Vitamin B-6	0.9 mg	Phosphorus	271.3 mg
Vitamin B-12	1.5 µg	Magnesium	77.4 mg
Folate (total)	36.6 µg	Zinc	1.3 mg
Vitamin C	34.7 mg	Potassium	1,141.5 mg

Dane's Tuna Casserole

PER SERVING: 259.9 CALORIES — 28.0 g PROTEIN — 22.9 g CARBOHYDRATE — 2.2 g FIBER —
5.6 g TOTAL FAT — 2.3 g SATURATED FAT — 88.9 mg CHOLESTEROL — 730.8 mg SODIUM

2 cans (6 ounces each) water-packed tuna, drained, finely flaked
1 cup cooked brown or white rice
1 small onion, very finely chopped
1 cup celery, very finely chopped
$^{1}/_{2}$ cup green bell pepper, very finely chopped
1 can (10$^{3}/_{4}$ ounces) reduced-sodium,
reduced-fat cream of mushroom soup (condensed)
1 egg, lightly beaten
1 tablespoon lemon juice
$^{1}/_{4}$–$^{1}/_{2}$ cup (1–2 ounces) grated Parmesan cheese

Combine all ingredients, except Parmesan cheese, in large
bowl, mixing well. Spoon into lightly greased 1$^{1}/_{2}$-quart casserole.
Sprinkle with cheese. Bake, uncovered, at 350 degrees until hot
and bubbly, about 35 minutes.

Makes 4 servings.

Nutritional Analysis per Serving

Vitamin A	62.7 RE	Vitamin D	0.2 µg
Thiamin (B-1)	0.1 mg	Vitamin E	1.0 mg
Riboflavin (B-2)	0.2 mg	Calcium	192.1 mg
Niacin	12.6 mg	Iron	2.0 mg
Vitamin B-6	0.5 mg	Phosphorus	262.0 mg
Vitamin B-12	2.7 µg	Magnesium	55.9 mg
Folate (total)	29.8 µg	Zinc	1.4 mg
Vitamin C	22.2 mg	Potassium	689.3 mg

Tuna–Mac Casserole

PER SERVING: 579.9 CALORIES — 37.2 g PROTEIN — 61.0 g CARBOHYDRATE — 2.9 g FIBER —
20.1 g TOTAL FAT — 12.2 g SATURATED FAT — 74.0 mg CHOLESTEROL — 1,015.4 mg SODIUM

8 ounces small macaroni, cooked

$1/2$ medium green bell pepper, finely chopped

1 can ($10^{3}/4$ ounces) tomato soup (condensed)

1 can (6 ounces) evaporated fat-free milk

$1/4$ cup water

1 can (6 ounces) water-packed tuna, drained, finely flaked

2 cups (8 ounces) shredded Cheddar cheese, divided

Combine macaroni, bell pepper, tomato soup, milk, water, tuna, and $1^{1}/2$ cup cheese in lightly greased 2-quart casserole. Sprinkle remaining $1/2$ cup cheese over top. Bake, uncovered, at 350 degrees until bubbly and lightly browned, about 40 minutes.

Makes 4 servings.

Nutritional Analysis per Serving

Vitamin A	261.4 RE	Vitamin D	1.1 µg
Thiamin (B-1)	0.5 mg	Vitamin E	0.6 mg
Riboflavin (B-2)	0.6 mg	Calcium	574.6 mg
Niacin	9.1 mg	Iron	3.3 mg
Vitamin B-6	0.3 mg	Phosphorus	527.2 mg
Vitamin B-12	1.9 µg	Magnesium	64.9 mg
Folate (total)	111.3 µg	Zinc	3.2 mg
Vitamin C	15.4 mg	Potassium	369.0 mg

Tuna Paté

PER SERVING: 228.6 CALORIES — 18.3 g PROTEIN — 0.5 g CARBOHYDRATE — 0.1 g FIBER —
16.9 g TOTAL FAT — 10.3 g SATURATED FAT — 80.0 mg CHOLESTEROL — 390.9 mg SODIUM

2 cans (6 ounces each) water-packed tuna, drained
1 stick butter or margarine, softened
1–2 teaspoons lemon juice
10 medium shrimp, cooked, shelled
3 tablespoons finely chopped pimentos
Hot pepper sauce, to taste
Salt and pepper, to taste

Process tuna, butter, and lemon juice in food processor until smooth. Add shrimp and pimentos. Process until finely chopped. Season to taste with hot pepper sauce, salt, and pepper. Spoon into small bowl. Refrigerate, covered, until chilled.

Serve spread over soft bread**

**Nutritional information does not include the bread accompaniment

Nutritional Analysis per Serving

Vitamin A	183.5 RE	Vitamin D	0.7 µg
Thiamin (B-1)	0.0 mg	Vitamin E	0.8 mg
Riboflavin (B-2)	0.1 mg	Calcium	18.0 mg
Niacin	8.5 mg	Iron	1.4 mg
Vitamin B-6	0.2 mg	Phosphorus	129.7 mg
Vitamin B-12	2.0 µg	Magnesium	21.7 mg
Folate (total)	3.9 µg	Zinc	0.6 mg
Vitamin C	5.7 mg	Potassium	182.9 mg

Broiled Turkey Burgers

PER SERVING: 209.7 CALORIES — 22.2 g PROTEIN — 5.3 g CARBOHYDRATE — 0.5 g FIBER —
10.5 g TOTAL FAT — 2.9 g SATURATED FAT — 125.1 mg CHOLESTEROL — 652.7 mg SODIUM

1 1/2 pounds twice-ground lean turkey

1/4 cup seasoned dry bread crumbs

1/4 cup finely chopped mushrooms

1/4 cup finely chopped green onion

2 garlic cloves, minced

1 1/2 teaspoons ground ginger

2 1/2 tablespoons soy sauce

1 egg, lightly beaten

Mix all ingredients in large bowl until well blended. Shape into six patties. Broil, 6 inches from heat source, until juices run clear, about 5 minutes on each side.

Makes 6 servings.

Nutritional Analysis per Serving

Vitamin A	19.5 RE	Vitamin D	0.2 µg
Thiamin (B-1)	0.1 mg	Vitamin E	0.5 mg
Riboflavin (B-2)	0.2 mg	Calcium	25.0 mg
Niacin	4.1 mg	Iron	1.9 mg
Vitamin B-6	0.3 mg	Phosphorus	178.0 mg
Vitamin B-12	0.3 µg	Magnesium	24.7 mg
Folate (total)	18.6 µg	Zinc	2.4 mg
Vitamin C	1.2 mg	Potassium	267.6 mg

Curried Turkey Casserole

PER SERVING: 273.6 CALORIES — 26.9 g PROTEIN — 11.4 g CARBOHYDRATE — 1.5 g FIBER — 12.6 g TOTAL FAT — 4.4 g SATURATED FAT — 73.3 mg CHOLESTEROL — 604.4 mg SODIUM

1 package (10 ounces) frozen chopped broccoli, thawed, drained

4 cups finely chopped cooked turkey

1 can (10³/₄ ounces) reduced-sodium,
reduced-fat cream of celery soup (condensed)

1 can (10³/₄ ounces) reduced-sodium,
reduced-fat cream of mushroom soup (condensed)

³/₄ cup fat-free milk

¹/₂ cup reduced-fat mayonnaise

1–2 teaspoons curry powder

1 tablespoon lemon juice

1 cup (4 ounces) shredded reduced-fat mild Cheddar cheese

Layer broccoli and turkey in lightly greased 9 x 13-inch baking pan. Blend remaining ingredients, except cheese, in medium bowl and pour over turkey; sprinkle with cheese. Bake, uncovered, at 350 degrees, 45 to 60 minutes, or until hot and bubbly.

Makes 8 servings.

Nutritional Analysis per Serving

Vitamin A	141.8 RE	Vitamin D	0.2 µg
Thiamin (B-1)	0.1 mg	Vitamin E	1.4 mg
Riboflavin (B-2)	0.3 mg	Calcium	247.3 mg
Niacin	4.1 mg	Iron	1.6 mg
Vitamin B-6	0.4 mg	Phosphorus	274.1 mg
Vitamin B-12	0.5 µg	Magnesium	32.2 mg
Folate (total)	31.5 µg	Zinc	3.1 mg
Vitamin C	22.0 mg	Potassium	499.8 mg

Turkey and Broccoli Tetrazzini

PER SERVING: 446.7 CALORIES — 29.5 g PROTEIN — 48.2 g CARBOHYDRATE — 2.8 g FIBER —
14.4 g TOTAL FAT — 3.4 g SATURATED FAT — 57.5 mg CHOLESTEROL — 723.9 mg SODIUM

$3/4$ cup reduced-fat mayonnaise

$1/3$ cup all-purpose flour

2 tablespoons minced onion

1 teaspoon garlic salt

$2^{1}/4$ cups fat-free milk

1 cup (4 ounces) shredded reduced-fat Swiss cheese

8 ounces thin spaghetti, cooked, drained, finely chopped

2 cups finely chopped cooked turkey breast

1 package (10 ounces) frozen broccoli, thawed, drained, finely chopped

$1/4$ cup chopped pimiento

1 can ($10^{3}/4$ ounces) reduced-sodium,
reduced-fat cream of mushroom soup (condensed)

Blend mayonnaise, flour, minced onion, and garlic salt in large saucepan. Add milk and cook over medium heat until thick, stirring constantly. Add cheese, stirring over low heat until melted. Stir in remaining ingredients. Spoon into lightly greased 9 x 13-inch baking dish. Bake, uncovered, at 350 degrees until hot and bubbly, about 30 minutes.

Makes 6 servings.

Nutritional Analysis per Serving

Vitamin A	195.2 RE	Vitamin D	0.9 µg
Thiamin (B-1)	0.4 mg	Vitamin E	2.3 mg
Riboflavin (B-2)	0.5 mg	Calcium	375.7 mg
Niacin	5.3 mg	Iron	2.9 mg
Vitamin B-6	0.4 mg	Phosphorus	396.8 mg
Vitamin B-12	0.9 µg	Magnesium	55.2 mg
Folate (total)	104.2 µg	Zinc	3.3 mg
Vitamin C	28.0 mg	Potassium	646.0 mg

Skillet Sausage and Tomatoes

PER SERVING: 183.2 CALORIES — 15.2 g PROTEIN — 9.1 g CARBOHYDRATE — 1.9 g FIBER —
10.3 g TOTAL FAT — 3.7 g SATURATED FAT — 65.3 mg CHOLESTEROL — 578.7 mg SODIUM

1 pound twice-ground turkey or pork sausage

1 medium onion, finely chopped

$1/2$ green bell pepper, finely chopped

1 can (15 ounces) reduced-sodium Italian-seasoned tomatoes,
undrained, finely chopped

$1/2$ cup tomato juice

1–2 teaspoons chili powder

$1/2$–1 cup reduced-fat sour cream

Salt and pepper, to taste

Cook sausage, onion, and pepper in large skillet over medium-high heat until sausage is browned, about 8 minutes, crumbling sausage finely with fork; drain fat. Add remaining ingredients, except sour cream. Heat to boiling; reduce heat and simmer, covered, 20 minutes. Add sour cream, stirring over low heat until hot. Season to taste with salt and pepper.

Makes 6 servings.

Nutritional Analysis per Serving

Vitamin A	100.9 RE	Vitamin D	0.0 µg
Thiamin (B-1)	0.0 mg	Vitamin E	0.3 mg
Riboflavin (B-2)	0.1 mg	Calcium	101.5 mg
Niacin	0.2 mg	Iron	1.6 mg
Vitamin B-6	0.1 mg	Phosphorus	39.8 mg
Vitamin B-12	0.1 µg	Magnesium	5.8 mg
Folate (total)	10.2 µg	Zinc	0.1 mg
Vitamin C	19.1 mg	Potassium	146.0 mg

Egg and Sausage Casserole

PER SERVING: 305.8 CALORIES — 18.9 g PROTEIN — 5.1 g CARBOHYDRATE — 0.0 g FIBER —
23.5 g TOTAL FAT — 9.0 g SATURATED FAT — 358.3 mg CHOLESTEROL — 600.5 mg SODIUM

12 ounces turkey breakfast sausage

12 eggs, lightly scrambled

1 can (10³/₄ ounces) reduced-sodium, reduced-fat
cream of mushroom soup (condensed)

¹/₂ cup fat-free milk

1 cup (4 ounces) shredded reduced-fat Cheddar cheese

Cook sausage in large skillet over medium-high heat until
browned, about 8 minutes, crumbling finely with fork; drain fat.
Spoon sausage into greased 1¹/₂-quart casserole; top with eggs.
Combine mushroom soup, milk, and cheese in medium bowl;
pour over eggs. Bake, uncovered, at 350 degrees until lightly
browned, about 20 minutes.

Makes 8 servings.

Nutritional Analysis per Serving

Vitamin A	206.3 RE	Vitamin D	1.1 µg
Thiamin (B-1)	0.1 mg	Vitamin E	0.8 mg
Riboflavin (B-2)	0.5 mg	Calcium	196.0 mg
Niacin	0.2 mg	Iron	1.4 mg
Vitamin B-6	0.1 mg	Phosphorus	224.0 mg
Vitamin B-12	0.9 µg	Magnesium	13.2 mg
Folate (total)	36.0 µg	Zinc	1.5 mg
Vitamin C	0.7 mg	Potassium	278.3 mg

Chicken and Mushroom Casserole

PER SERVING: 316.0 CALORIES — 32.4 g PROTEIN — 22.8 g CARBOHYDRATE — 2.1 g FIBER —
9.3 g TOTAL FAT — 4.0 g SATURATED FAT — 88.6 mg CHOLESTEROL — 606.8 mg SODIUM

1 1/2 pounds cooked chicken breast, finely chopped

2 cups reduced-fat sour cream

1 can (10 3/4 ounces) reduced-sodium, reduced-fat
cream of mushroom soup (condensed)

1 teaspoon Worcestershire sauce

1 can (4 ounces) mushrooms, drained, finely chopped

1 package (6 ounces) chicken-flavored stuffing mix

Place chicken in lightly greased 9 x 13-inch baking pan. Mix
sour cream, mushroom soup, Worcestershire sauce, and mushrooms. Pour over chicken. Prepare stuffing mix according to
package directions; spread over casserole. Bake, loosely covered,
at 350 degrees or until hot and lightly browned, about 30 minutes.

Makes 8 servings.

Nutritional Analysis per Serving

Vitamin A	125.1 RE	Vitamin D	0.0 µg
Thiamin (B-1)	0.2 mg	Vitamin E	0.2 mg
Riboflavin (B-2)	0.3 mg	Calcium	182.1 mg
Niacin	8.7 mg	Iron	1.7 mg
Vitamin B-6	0.3 mg	Phosphorus	222.7 mg
Vitamin B-12	0.4 µg	Magnesium	20.4 mg
Folate (total)	2.6 µg	Zinc	0.8 mg
Vitamin C	0.0 mg	Potassium	473.6 mg

The Slick Chick

PER SERVING: 356.0 CALORIES — 31.0 g PROTEIN — 41.3 g CARBOHYDRATE — 2.8 g FIBER —
6.2 g TOTAL FAT — 2.4 g SATURATED FAT — 64.4 mg CHOLESTEROL — 615.0 mg SODIUM

1 can (10³/₄ ounces) reduced-sodium, reduced-fat
cream of mushroom soup (condensed)

1 can (10³/₄ ounces) reduced-sodium, reduced-fat
cream of chicken soup (condensed)

¹/₂ cup fat-free milk

1 teaspoon onion powder

4 cups cooked brown or white rice

3 cups finely chopped cooked chicken breast

1 cup (4 ounces) shredded reduced-fat Cheddar cheese

2 tablespoons finely chopped pimento

Combine soups and milk in large saucepan; heat to simmering, stirring frequently. Stir in remaining ingredients. Pour into
lightly greased 2-quart casserole. Bake, uncovered, at 375 until
lightly browned, about 30 minutes.

Makes 6 servings.

Nutritional Analysis per Serving

Vitamin A	109.6 RE	Vitamin D	0.3 µg
Thiamin (B-1)	0.2 mg	Vitamin E	0.5 mg
Riboflavin (B-2)	0.2 mg	Calcium	157.7 mg
Niacin	8.3 mg	Iron	1.2 mg
Vitamin B-6	0.4 mg	Phosphorus	245.8 mg
Vitamin B-12	0.2 µg	Magnesium	75.6 mg
Folate (total)	9.1 µg	Zinc	1.6 mg
Vitamin C	13.8 mg	Potassium	416.5 mg

Chicken Noodle Casserole

PER SERVING: 472.1 CALORIES — 37.2 g PROTEIN — 47.0 g CARBOHYDRATE — 2.1 g FIBER — 14.9 g TOTAL FAT — 7.8 g SATURATED FAT — 134.4 mg CHOLESTEROL — 631.4 mg SODIUM

6 ounces thin egg noodles, cooked

1 can (10¾ ounces) reduced-sodium, reduced-fat cream of chicken soup (condensed)

1 can (6 ounces) evaporated milk

1 cup (4 ounces) shredded reduced-fat American cheese

2 cups finely chopped cooked chicken breast

1 cup very finely chopped celery

¼ cup very finely chopped green bell pepper

¼ cup finely chopped pimentos

Spoon noodles into lightly greased 2-quart casserole. Combine chicken soup and evaporated milk in medium saucepan; heat to simmering, stirring frequently. Add cheese, stirring over low heat until melted. Stir in remaining ingredients; pour over noodles. Bake, uncovered, at 350 degrees until lightly browned and bubbly, about 30 minutes.

Makes 4 servings.

Nutritional Analysis per Serving

Vitamin A	202.2 RE	Vitamin D	0.9 µg
Thiamin (B-1)	0.4 mg	Vitamin E	0.5 mg
Riboflavin (B-2)	0.4 mg	Calcium	408.5 mg
Niacin	8.7 mg	Iron	2.5 mg
Vitamin B-6	0.4 mg	Phosphorus	300.2 mg
Vitamin B-12	0.4 µg	Magnesium	54.8 mg
Folate (total)	85.9 µg	Zinc	1.8 mg
Vitamin C	36.7 mg	Potassium	425.4 mg

Chicken Encore

PER SERVING: 605.7 CALORIES — 50.3 g PROTEIN — 61.5 g CARBOHYDRATE — 1.9 g FIBER —
15.9 g TOTAL FAT — 6.0 g SATURATED FAT — 309.4 mg CHOLESTEROL — 980.9 mg SODIUM

12 ounces cooked chicken, finely chopped

8 ounces uncooked, very small elbow macaroni

2 cans (10³/₄ ounces each) reduced-sodium, reduced-fat
cream of mushroom soup (condensed)

4 hard-cooked eggs, finely chopped

1 medium onion, finely chopped

1 cup fat-free milk

1 cup reduced-sodium, fat-free chicken broth

1–1¹/₂ cups (4–6 ounces) shredded reduced-fat Monterey Jack or mozzarella cheese

Combine all ingredients in 9 x 13–inch baking dish, mixing
well. Cover and refrigerate overnight. Bake, covered, at 350 degrees
until macaroni is tender, about 1 hour.

Makes 4 servings.

Nutritional Analysis per Serving

Vitamin A	228.1 RE	Vitamin D	1.3 µg
Thiamin (B-1)	0.5 mg	Vitamin E	0.9 mg
Riboflavin (B-2)	0.8 mg	Calcium	440.8 mg
Niacin	10.6 mg	Iron	3.2 mg
Vitamin B-6	0.5 mg	Phosphorus	522.8 mg
Vitamin B-12	1.3 µg	Magnesium	64.1 mg
Folate (total)	126.2 µg	Zinc	3.3 mg
Vitamin C	2.4 mg	Potassium	969.4 mg

Baked Chicken Salad

PER SERVING: 303.6 CALORIES — 32.7 g PROTEIN — 12.4 g CARBOHYDRATE — 1.3 g FIBER —
12.5 g TOTAL FAT — 3.8 g SATURATED FAT — 182.4 mg CHOLESTEROL — 551.2 mg SODIUM

1 cup finely crushed potato chips
³/₄ cup (3 ounces) shredded reduced-fat Cheddar cheese, divided
1¹/₂ pounds cooked chicken breast, finely chopped
1 cup finely chopped celery
2 tablespoons finely chopped onion
¹/₄ cup finely chopped pimentos
³/₄ cup fat-free mayonnaise
1 can (10³/₄ ounces) reduced-sodium, reduced-fat
cream of chicken soup (condensed)
¹/₃ cup finely chopped almonds
2 tablespoons lemon juice
4 hard-cooked eggs, finely chopped

Mix potato chips and cheese in small bowl. Combine half the potato chip mixture and remaining ingredients, except eggs, in large bowl. Spoon into lightly greased 2¹/₂-quart baking dish. Sprinkle with eggs; top with remaining potato chip mixture. Refrigerate, covered, several hours or overnight. Bake, covered, at 350 degrees until browned and bubbly, about 25 minutes.

Makes 8 servings.

Nutritional Analysis per Serving

Vitamin A	136.4 RE	Vitamin D	0.3 µg
Thiamin (B-1)	0.1 mg	Vitamin E	2.6 mg
Riboflavin (B-2)	0.3 mg	Calcium	120.0 mg
Niacin	7.8 mg	Iron	1.6 mg
Vitamin B-6	0.4 mg	Phosphorus	280.7 mg
Vitamin B-12	0.5 µg	Magnesium	46.6 mg
Folate (total)	23.7 µg	Zinc	1.8 mg
Vitamin C	17.2 mg	Potassium	385.5 mg

Onion–Cheddar Bake

PER SERVING: 207.7 CALORIES — 14.7 g PROTEIN — 10.4 g CARBOHYDRATE — 1.7 g FIBER — 11.2 g TOTAL FAT — 5.6 g SATURATED FAT — 232.8 mg CHOLESTEROL — 523.5 mg SODIUM

4 medium onions, finely chopped
1 medium green bell pepper, finely chopped
1¹/₂ cups (6 ounces) shredded reduced-fat Cheddar cheese
6 eggs
¹/₃ cup fat-free milk
2 tablespoons Worcestershire sauce
¹/₂ teaspoon salt
¹/₄ teaspoon pepper

Cook onions and bell pepper in medium saucepan in lightly salted boiling water 5 minutes. Drain; place half the onion mixture in lightly greased 7 x 11-inch baking dish. Sprinkle with half the cheese. Repeat with remaining onion mixture and cheese. Beat eggs, milk, Worcestershire sauce, salt, and pepper in medium bowl; pour over cheese. Bake, uncovered, at 350 degrees until lightly browned and set, about 30 minutes.

Makes 6 servings.

Nutritional Analysis per Serving

Vitamin A	206.3 RE	Vitamin D	0.8 µg
Thiamin (B-1)	0.1 mg	Vitamin E	0.8 mg
Riboflavin (B-2)	0.4 mg	Calcium	262.2 mg
Niacin	0.3 mg	Iron	1.1 mg
Vitamin B-6	0.2 mg	Phosphorus	281.2 mg
Vitamin B-12	0.8 µg	Magnesium	24.0 mg
Folate (total)	42.5 µg	Zinc	2.0 mg
Vitamin C	22.6 mg	Potassium	292.4 mg

Spinach–Cheese Pie

PER SERVING: 553.8 CALORIES — 31.6 g PROTEIN — 22.9 g CARBOHYDRATE — 3.4 g FIBER — 37.9 g TOTAL FAT — 19.2 g SATURATED FAT — 172.9 mg CHOLESTEROL — 1,243.9 mg SODIUM

4 cups (16 ounces) shredded provolone cheese
1 prepared 9-inch, deep-dish pie crust
2 packages (10 ounces each) frozen chopped spinach, thawed, well drained
3 eggs, lightly beaten
$1/2$ cup reduced-fat sour cream
$1/2$ teaspoon salt
$1/4$ teaspoon pepper

Arrange cheese in a 9-inch, deep-dish pie crust. Combine remaining ingredients; spoon into pie crust. Bake, uncovered, at 325 degrees until browned and sharp knife inserted halfway between center and edge comes out clean, about 45 minutes.
Makes 6 servings.

Nutritional Analysis per Serving

Vitamin A	1,052.4 RE	Vitamin D	0.3 µg
Thiamin (B-1)	0.2 mg	Vitamin E	1.5 mg
Riboflavin (B-2)	0.7 mg	Calcium	850.8 mg
Niacin	1.5 mg	Iron	3.1 mg
Vitamin B-6	0.2 mg	Phosphorus	567.9 mg
Vitamin B-12	1.6 µg	Magnesium	96.4 mg
Folate (total)	142.6 µg	Zinc	3.9 mg
Vitamin C	11.6 mg	Potassium	499.7 mg

Lamb Loaves

PER SERVING: 282.4 CALORIES — 23.9 g PROTEIN — 11.1 g CARBOHYDRATE — 0.9 g FIBER —
15.4 g TOTAL FAT — 5.9 g SATURATED FAT — 74.3 mg CHOLESTEROL — 585.8 mg SODIUM

1 pound twice-ground lean lamb leg

$1/2$ pound twice-ground lean beef

2 cups fresh white bread crumbs

1 can ($10^3/4$ ounces) onion soup (condensed)

1 teaspoon dried oregano leaves

$1/2$ teaspoon dried mint leaves

$1/2$ teaspoon pepper

Mix all ingredients; shape into loaf in 9 x 13-inch baking pan.
Bake at 350 degrees until loaf is no longer pink in the center,
about 1 hour.

Makes 6 servings.

NOTE: Meat mixture can also be pressed lightly into
12 muffin cups. Bake at 350 degrees until no longer pink in
the center, 15 to 20 minutes.

Nutritional Analysis per Serving

Vitamin A	2.2 RE	Vitamin D	0.0 µg
Thiamin (B-1)	0.1 mg	Vitamin E	0.4 mg
Riboflavin (B-2)	0.3 mg	Calcium	41.4 mg
Niacin	6.9 mg	Iron	3.0 mg
Vitamin B-6	0.2 mg	Phosphorus	205.2 mg
Vitamin B-12	2.0 µg	Magnesium	31.6 mg
Folate (total)	33.2 µg	Zinc	4.5 mg
Vitamin C	0.7 mg	Potassium	355.9 mg

Orange Lamb Patties

PER SERVING: 255.9 CALORIES — 23.2 g PROTEIN — 8.7 g CARBOHYDRATE — 0.5 g FIBER — 13.6 g TOTAL FAT — 5.5 g SATURATED FAT — 108.5 mg CHOLESTEROL — 586.2 mg SODIUM

1 1/2 pounds twice-ground lean lamb leg
1/4 cup unseasoned dry bread crumbs
1 egg
1 1/2 teaspoons ground coriander
2–3 teaspoons finely grated orange peel
1/4 cup orange juice concentrate
1–2 tablespoons reduced-sodium soy sauce
1 teaspoon salt
1/2 teaspoon pepper

Mix all ingredients; shape into 6 patties. Broil 6 inches from heat source to desired degree of doneness, about 5 minutes on each side.

Makes 6 servings.

Nutritional Analysis per Serving

Vitamin A	19.6 RE	Vitamin D	0.1 µg
Thiamin (B-1)	0.1 mg	Vitamin E	0.4 mg
Riboflavin (B-2)	0.3 mg	Calcium	32.8 mg
Niacin	7.1 mg	Iron	2.4 mg
Vitamin B-6	0.2 mg	Phosphorus	227.1 mg
Vitamin B-12	2.2 µg	Magnesium	34.6 mg
Folate (total)	42.1 µg	Zinc	4.1 mg
Vitamin C	17.3 mg	Potassium	402.1 mg

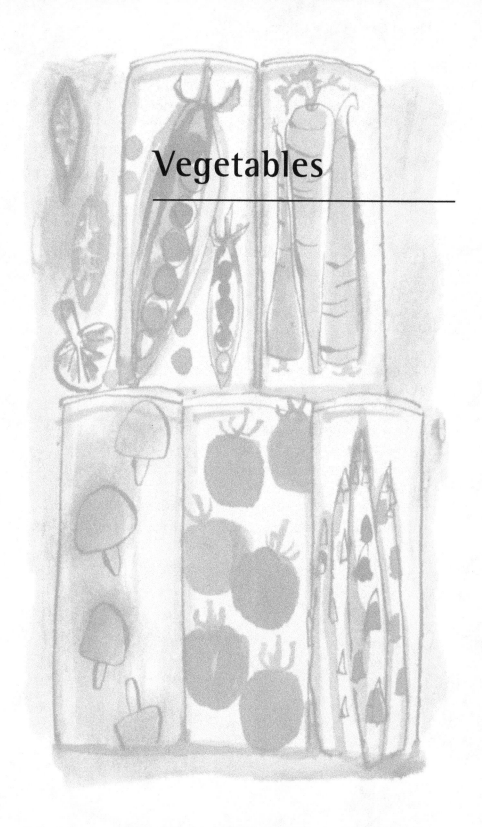

Vegetables

Egg and Asparagus Casserole

PER SERVING: 358.5 CALORIES — 18.6 g PROTEIN — 34.5 g CARBOHYDRATE — 4.6 g FIBER —
17.5 g TOTAL FAT — 8.5 g SATURATED FAT — 243.0 mg CHOLESTEROL — 695.7 mg SODIUM

3 slices whole wheat bread, cut into scant ¹/₂-inch cubes

12 ounces asparagus tips, cooked, drained, and finely chopped

4 hard-cooked eggs, finely chopped

2 tablespoons butter or margarine

2 tablespoons flour

1¹/₂ cups 1% low-fat milk

¹/₂ cup (2 ounces) shredded reduced-fat American cheese

Salt and pepper, to taste

¹/₄ cup seasoned dry bread crumbs

¹/₄ cup finely chopped parsley

Layer bread cubes, asparagus, and eggs into greased 1¹/₂-quart casserole.

Melt butter in small saucepan; stir in flour and cook over medium heat, stirring constantly, 1 to 2 minutes. Stir in milk and heat to boiling; reduce heat and simmer until thickened, 1 to 2 minutes. Add cheese, stirring until melted; season to taste with salt and pepper.

Pour cheese sauce over ingredients in casserole. Sprinkle top with combined bread crumbs and parsley. Bake, uncovered, at 350 until hot through, 20 to 30 minutes.

Makes 4 servings.

Nutritional Analysis per Serving

Vitamin A	319.9 RE	Vitamin D	1.7 µg
Thiamin (B-1)	0.3 mg	Vitamin E	2.9 mg
Riboflavin (B-2)	0.6 mg	Calcium	312.1 mg
Niacin	2.7 mg	Iron	3.1 mg
Vitamin B-6	0.3 mg	Phosphorus	314.7 mg
Vitamin B-12	0.9 µg	Magnesium	71.1 mg
Folate (total)	151.9 µg	Zinc	2.0 mg
Vitamin C	15.6 mg	Potassium	607.1 mg

Favorite Broccoli Casserole

PER SERVING: 140.8 CALORIES — 6.0 g PROTEIN — 18.8 g CARBOHYDRATE — 2.0 g FIBER — 4.9 g TOTAL FAT — 2.8 g SATURATED FAT — 13.1 mg CHOLESTEROL — 434.4 mg SODIUM

1 package (10 ounces) frozen chopped broccoli, thawed and drained

$1/2$–1 cup (2 to 4 ounces) shredded reduced-fat Cheddar or mozzarella cheese

1 can ($10^3/4$ ounces) reduced-sodium, reduced-fat
cream of mushroom soup (condensed)

1 cup cooked rice

$1/2$ cup finely chopped onion

$1/4$ cup seasoned dry bread crumbs

1–2 tablespoons melted butter or margarine

Combine all ingredients, except bread crumbs and butter, in 2-quart greased casserole. Sprinkle combined bread crumbs and butter over the top. Bake, uncovered, at 350 degrees, until hot through, about 30 minutes.

Makes 6 servings.

Nutritional Analysis per Serving

Vitamin A	147.0 RE	Vitamin D	0.1 µg
Thiamin (B-1)	0.1 mg	Vitamin E	0.8 mg
Riboflavin (B-2)	0.1 mg	Calcium	161.6 mg
Niacin	0.9 mg	Iron	0.9 mg
Vitamin B-6	0.1 mg	Phosphorus	44.2 mg
Vitamin B-12	0.0 µg	Magnesium	14.5 mg
Folate (total)	43.9 µg	Zinc	0.4 mg
Vitamin C	20.9 mg	Potassium	320.7 mg

Party Broccoli Casserole

PER SERVING: 174.0 CALORIES — 10.3 g PROTEIN — 18.0 g CARBOHYDRATE — 4.3 g FIBER —
7.5 g TOTAL FAT — 4.0 g SATURATED FAT — 24.1 mg CHOLESTEROL — 386.6 mg SODIUM

3 packages (10 ounces each) frozen chopped broccoli, cooked and drained
1 jar (2 ounces) chopped pimentos
1 can (4 ounces) mushroom pieces, drained, finely chopped
1 can (10³/₄ ounces) reduced-sodium, reduced-fat
cream of mushroom soup (condensed)
2 containers (8 ounces) reduced-fat sour cream
2 cups fresh whole wheat bread crumbs
¹/₂ cup (2 ounces) shredded reduced-fat Cheddar cheese

Combine broccoli, pimentos, mushrooms, mushroom soup, and sour cream in greased 2-quart casserole. Toss bread crumbs and cheese; sprinkle over casserole. Bake, uncovered, at 350 degrees until hot through, about 30 minutes.

Makes 8 servings.

Nutritional Analysis per Serving

Vitamin A	357.3 RE	Vitamin D	0.0 µg
Thiamin (B-1)	0.1 mg	Vitamin E	1.8 mg
Riboflavin (B-2)	0.3 mg	Calcium	266.4 mg
Niacin	1.1 mg	Iron	1.3 mg
Vitamin B-6	0.2 mg	Phosphorus	147.5 mg
Vitamin B-12	0.2 µg	Magnesium	28.9 mg
Folate (total)	50.3 µg	Zinc	0.7 mg
Vitamin C	51.0 mg	Potassium	554.6 mg

Mexican Broccoli Bake

PER SERVING: 372.5 CALORIES — 26.8 g PROTEIN — 34.1 g CARBOHYDRATE — 4.9 g FIBER —
15.2 g TOTAL FAT — 7.7 g SATURATED FAT — 237.3 mg CHOLESTEROL — 839.8 mg SODIUM

1 package (10 ounces) frozen chopped broccoli, thawed and drained
4 eggs, beaten
2 cups 2% reduced-fat milk
2 cups cooked brown rice
1–1 1/2 cups (4–6 ounces) shredded reduced-fat Cheddar cheese
1 can (4 ounces) mild green chilies, drained and finely chopped
1/2 teaspoon salt
1/2 teaspoon pepper

Combine all ingredients in a greased 2-quart casserole. Bake, uncovered, at 350 degrees until puffed and browned, 30 to 40 minutes. Let stand 10 minutes before serving.

Makes 4 servings.

Nutritional Analysis per Serving

Vitamin A	477.1 RE	Vitamin D	2.0 µg
Thiamin (B-1)	0.2 mg	Vitamin E	1.9 mg
Riboflavin (B-2)	0.5 mg	Calcium	634.9 mg
Niacin	1.9 mg	Iron	1.8 mg
Vitamin B-6	0.3 mg	Phosphorus	318.2 mg
Vitamin B-12	0.9 µg	Magnesium	76.6 mg
Folate (total)	64.4 µg	Zinc	2.0 mg
Vitamin C	36.9 mg	Potassium	428.9 mg

Broccoli–Brown Rice Casserole

PER SERVING: 181.9 CALORIES — 7.5 g PROTEIN — 25.1 g CARBOHYDRATE — 3.4 g FIBER —
6.1 g TOTAL FAT — 3.2 g SATURATED FAT — 17.3 mg CHOLESTEROL — 517.9 mg SODIUM

1/4 cup finely chopped onion

1/4 cup finely chopped celery

1–2 tablespoons butter or margarine

1 can (10 3/4 ounces) reduced-sodium, reduced-fat
cream of chicken soup (condensed)

1 can (10 3/4 ounces) reduced-sodium, reduced-fat
cream of mushroom soup (condensed)

1/2–1 cup (2–4 ounces) shredded reduced-fat Cheddar cheese

1 package (16 ounces) frozen chopped broccoli, thawed and drained

1 1/2 cups cooked brown rice

Sauté onion and celery in butter in small skillet until tender,
2 to 3 minutes. Combine onion and celery mixture and remaining
ingredients in greased 1 1/2-quart casserole. Bake, covered, at 350
degrees until hot through, about 30 minutes.

Makes 6 servings.

Nutritional Analysis per Serving

Vitamin A	242.7 RE	Vitamin D	0.1 µg
Thiamin (B-1)	0.1 mg	Vitamin E	1.3 mg
Riboflavin (B-2)	0.1 mg	Calcium	174.7 mg
Niacin	1.4 mg	Iron	0.8 mg
Vitamin B-6	0.2 mg	Phosphorus	78.5 mg
Vitamin B-12	0.0 µg	Magnesium	35.2 mg
Folate (total)	37.6 µg	Zinc	0.7 mg
Vitamin C	42.9 mg	Potassium	376.9 mg

Brussels Sprout Soufflé

PER SERVING: 180.1 CALORIES — 10.3 g PROTEIN — 15.3 g CARBOHYDRATE — 3.4 g FIBER —
9.3 g TOTAL FAT — 4.5 g SATURATED FAT — 174.9 mg CHOLESTEROL — 471.5 mg SODIUM

1 tablespoon butter or margarine, softened	$^{1}/_{2}$ cup whole milk
3 tablespoons grated Parmesan cheese, divided	3 egg yolks
	$^{1}/_{2}$ teaspoon salt
10 ounces Brussels sprouts, trimmed, cooked	$^{1}/_{4}$ teaspoon pepper
	$^{1}/_{8}$ teaspoon ground nutmeg
1 medium potato, peeled, cubed, cooked	Dash hot pepper sauce
	3 egg whites, beaten to stiff peaks

Coat inside of 1-quart soufflé dish with the butter. Sprinkle 1 tablespoon of the Parmesan cheese over bottom and sides of dish. To make collar for soufflé, tear off a length of aluminum foil long enough to encircle dish. Fold in half lengthwise. Fasten collar to dish with string or tape so collar is 2 inches higher than rim.

Process Brussels sprouts, potato, and milk in food processor or blender until smooth; transfer to bowl. Beat egg yolks into Brussels-sprout mixture one at a time, beating well after each addition. Stir in remaining 2 tablespoons Parmesan cheese, salt, pepper, nutmeg, and hot pepper sauce. Fold beaten egg whites into Brussels sprout mixture until no streaks of white remain. Pour into prepared souffle dish.

Place soufflé in preheated 400 degree oven; immediately lower temperature to 375 degrees and bake, uncovered, until puffed and golden, about 35 minutes.

Makes 4 servings.

Nutritional Analysis per Serving

Vitamin A	173.1 RE	Vitamin D	0.8 µg
Thiamin (B-1)	0.1 mg	Vitamin E	1.2 mg
Riboflavin (B-2)	0.3 mg	Calcium	139.2 mg
Niacin	1.0 mg	Iron	1.6 mg
Vitamin B-6	0.3 mg	Phosphorus	181.5 mg
Vitamin B-12	0.6 µg	Magnesium	32.5 mg
Folate (total)	52.1 µg	Zinc	1.0 mg
Vitamin C	48.0 mg	Potassium	460.5 mg

Carrot–Rice Casserole

PER SERVING: 203.5 CALORIES — 11.0 g PROTEIN — 28.4 g CARBOHYDRATE — 2.7 g FIBER —
5.6 g TOTAL FAT — 3.3 g SATURATED FAT — 12.1 mg CHOLESTEROL — 522.6 mg SODIUM

2 cups water, divided

$1/4$ teaspoon salt

3 cups carrots, finely shredded

$2/3$ cup uncooked rice

$1^1/2$ cups (6 ounces) shredded reduced-fat Cheddar cheese, divided

1 can ($10^3/4$ ounces) reduced-sodium, reduced-fat cream of celery soup (condensed)

$1/4$ cup finely chopped onion

$1/4$ teaspoon dried thyme leaves

Heat $1^1/2$ cups water and salt to boiling in medium saucepan; add carrots and rice and simmer, covered, until rice is tender and water absorbed, about 20 minutes. Stir in $1^1/2$ cups cheese, celery soup, onion, thyme, and remaining $1/2$ cup water. Spoon into greased $1^1/2$-quart casserole. Bake, uncovered, at 350 degrees, 20 minutes, sprinkling with remaining $1/2$ cup cheese during last 5 minutes of baking time.

Makes 6 servings.

Nutritional Analysis per Serving

Vitamin A	1,827.6 RE	Vitamin D	0.1 µg
Thiamin (B-1)	0.2 mg	Vitamin E	0.3 mg
Riboflavin (B-2)	0 mg	Calcium	338.1 mg
Niacin	1.4 mg	Iron	1.3 mg
Vitamin B-6	0.1 mg	Phosphorus	52.7 mg
Vitamin B-12	0.0 µg	Magnesium	15.0 mg
Folate (total)	57.4 µg	Zinc	0.4 mg
Vitamin C	6.1 mg	Potassium	230.7 mg

Carrot Purée

PER SERVING: 90.9 CALORIES — 1.3 g PROTEIN — 15.0 g CARBOHYDRATE — 3.4 g FIBER —
3.4 g TOTAL FAT — 2.0 g SATURATED FAT — 8.7 mg CHOLESTEROL — 73.9 mg SODIUM

1 pound carrots, sliced, cooked, warm
1–2 tablespoons butter or margarine
1–2 tablespoons whole milk
1–2 tablespoons packed light brown sugar
Ground cinnamon, to taste
Ground nutmeg, to taste
Salt and pepper, to taste

Process carrots, butter, milk, and brown sugar in food processor or blender until smooth. Season to taste with cinnamon, nutmeg, salt, and pepper.

Makes 4 servings.

Nutritional Analysis per Serving

Vitamin A	2,900.4 RE	Vitamin D	0.1 µg
Thiamin (B-1)	0.1 mg	Vitamin E	0.6 mg
Riboflavin (B-2)	0.1 mg	Calcium	39.0 mg
Niacin	1.0 mg	Iron	0.6 mg
Vitamin B-6	0.2 mg	Phosphorus	55.1 mg
Vitamin B-12	0.0 µg	Magnesium	18.6 mg
Folate (total)	13.0 µg	Zinc	0.2 mg
Vitamin C	7.9 mg	Potassium	384.9 mg

Carrot Soufflé

PER SERVING: 78.9 CALORIES — 4.7 g PROTEIN — 7.5 g CARBOHYDRATE — 0.9 g FIBER —
3.3 g TOTAL FAT — 1.1 g SATURATED FAT — 108.0 mg CHOLESTEROL — 281.9 mg SODIUM

1 cup finely shredded carrots

1 cup fresh white bread crumbs

1/2 cup 2% reduced-fat milk

1/4 cup finely chopped onion

3 egg yolks

1/2 teaspoon salt

1/4 teaspoon pepper

3 egg whites, beaten to stiff peaks

Mix all ingredients, except egg whites. Fold egg whites into mixture; pour into ungreased 1-quart casserole. Bake, uncovered, at 350 degrees until set, about 30 minutes.

Makes 6 servings.

Nutritional Analysis per Serving

Vitamin A	575.8 RE	Vitamin D	0.5 µg
Thiamin (B-1)	0.1 mg	Vitamin E	0.4 mg
Riboflavin (B-2)	0.2 mg	Calcium	52.1 mg
Niacin	0.5 mg	Iron	0.7 mg
Vitamin B-6	0.1 mg	Phosphorus	79.5 mg
Vitamin B-12	0.4 µg	Magnesium	10.8 mg
Folate (total)	24.6 µg	Zinc	0.4 mg
Vitamin C	2.4 mg	Potassium	142.7 mg

Cauliflower Purée

PER SERVING: 64.0 CALORIES — 4.7 g PROTEIN — 6.0 g CARBOHYDRATE — 5.7 g FIBER —
3.6 g TOTAL FAT — 1.9 g SATURATED FAT — 8.2 mg CHOLESTEROL — 103.5 mg SODIUM

1 medium head cauliflower, cut into florets, cooked, warm
1–2 teaspoons lemon juice
1–2 tablespoons butter or margarine, cut into pieces
Ground nutmeg, to taste
Salt and pepper, to taste

Process cauliflower, lemon juice, and butter in food processor or blender until smooth. Season to taste with nutmeg, salt, and pepper.

Makes 4 servings.

Nutritional Analysis per Serving

Vitamin A	32.3 RE	Vitamin D	0.1 µg
Thiamin (B-1)	0.1 mg	Vitamin E	0.1 mg
Riboflavin (B-2)	0.2 mg	Calcium	47.5 mg
Niacin	1.2 mg	Iron	1.0 mg
Vitamin B-6	0.5 mg	Phosphorus	103.9 mg
Vitamin B-12	0.0 µg	Magnesium	37.2 mg
Folate (total)	0.4 µg	Zinc	0.6 mg
Vitamin C	149.6 mg	Potassium	658.1 mg

Corn Pudding

PER SERVING: 324.9 CALORIES — 11.7 g PROTEIN — 45.6 g CARBOHYDRATE — 2.7 g FIBER —
11.9 g TOTAL FAT — 4.7 g SATURATED FAT — 172.5 mg CHOLESTEROL — 803.2 mg SODIUM

1 can (16 ounces) creamed corn
1 cup fine saltine cracker crumbs
1 cup 2% reduced-fat milk
1/4 cup finely chopped green bell pepper
1 jar (2 ounces) pimentos, finely chopped
2 tablespoons finely chopped chives
1/4 teaspoon dry mustard
Salt and pepper, to taste
3 eggs, well beaten
1–2 tablespoons butter or margarine

Combine all ingredients, except salt, pepper, eggs, and butter in bowl, mixing well; season to taste with salt and pepper. Mix in eggs. Pour mixture into greased 1-quart casserole and dot with butter. Bake, uncovered, at 350 degrees until set, about 1 hour.

Makes 4 servings.

Nutritional Analysis per Serving

Vitamin A	196.1 RE	Vitamin D	1.2 µg
Thiamin (B-1)	0.2 mg	Vitamin E	1.2 mg
Riboflavin (B-2)	0.5 mg	Calcium	134.2 mg
Niacin	2.8 mg	Iron	2.8 mg
Vitamin B-6	0.2 mg	Phosphorus	218.2 mg
Vitamin B-12	0.6 µg	Magnesium	41.7 mg
Folate (total)	111.4 µg	Zinc	1.5 mg
Vitamin C	27.0 mg	Potassium	372.9 mg

Green Bean Delight

PER SERVING: 159.3 CALORIES — 6.5 g PROTEIN — 15.9 g CARBOHYDRATE — 3.1 g FIBER — 8.2 g TOTAL FAT — 4.9 g SATURATED FAT — 25.0 mg CHOLESTEROL — 354.0 mg SODIUM

$^1/_2$ cup finely chopped onion

1 tablespoon chopped parsley

2 tablespoons butter or margarine

5 cups cooked green beans, finely chopped

1 cup reduced-fat sour cream

$^1/_2$ cup shredded American cheese

$^1/_2$ cup bread crumbs

2 tablespoons flour

Salt and pepper, to taste

Sauté onion and parsley in butter until tender, about 3 minutes. Stir in flour and cook over medium heat 1 minute. Stir in sour cream and mix well; stir in green beans and season to taste with salt and pepper. Pour into lightly greased 2-quart baking dish; top with combined cheese and bread crumbs. Bake uncovered at 325 degrees 25 minutes or until hot through.

Makes 8 servings.

Nutritional Analysis per Serving

Vitamin A	163.6 RE	Vitamin D	0.1 µg
Thiamin (B-1)	0.1 mg	Vitamin E	0.2 mg
Riboflavin (B-2)	0.2 mg	Calcium	150.7 mg
Niacin	0.8 mg	Iron	1.4 mg
Vitamin B-6	0.1 mg	Phosphorus	139.6 mg
Vitamin B-12	0.2 µg	Magnesium	25.6 mg
Folate (total)	40.1 µg	Zinc	0.6 mg
Vitamin C	8.8 mg	Potassium	355.6 mg

Green Bean Casserole

PER SERVING: 156.0 CALORIES — 6.3 g PROTEIN — 16.3 g CARBOHYDRATE — 3.1 g FIBER — 7.7 g TOTAL FAT — 4.6 g SATURATED FAT — 22.8 mg CHOLESTEROL — 337.1 mg SODIUM

^{1}/$_2$ cup finely chopped onion

1 tablespoon chopped parsley

2 tablespoons butter or margarine

2 tablespoons flour

1 cup reduced-fat sour cream

5 cups cooked green beans, finely chopped

Salt and pepper, to taste

^{1}/$_2$ cup (2 ounces) shredded American cheese

^{1}/$_2$ cup seasoned dry bread crumbs

Sauté onion and parsley in butter until tender, about 3 minutes. Stir in flour and cook over medium heat, 1 minute. Stir in sour cream and mix well; stir in green beans and season to taste with salt and pepper. Pour into lightly greased 2-quart baking dish; top with combined cheese and bread crumbs. Bake uncovered at 325 degrees, 25 minutes or until hot through.

Makes 8 servings.

Nutritional Analysis per Serving

Vitamin A	158.6 RE	Vitamin D	0.1 µg
Thiamin (B-1)	0.1 mg	Vitamin E	0.2 mg
Riboflavin (B-2)	0.2 mg	Calcium	147.8 mg
Niacin	0.8 mg	Iron	1.4 mg
Vitamin B-6	0.1 mg	Phosphorus	119.4 mg
Vitamin B-12	0.2 µg	Magnesium	26.2 mg
Folate (total)	40.1 µg	Zinc	0.6 mg
Vitamin C	8.8 mg	Potassium	363.9 mg

Green Bean Puff-n-Stuff

PER SERVING: 207.9 CALORIES — 11.7 g PROTEIN — 14.8 g CARBOHYDRATE — 4.0 g FIBER — 12.2 g TOTAL FAT — 6.8 g SATURATED FAT — 132.6 mg CHOLESTEROL — 520.8 mg SODIUM

16 ounces fresh green beans, cooked, finely chopped
1 tablespoon minced onion
2 tablespoons butter or margarine
2 tablespoons flour
$^1/_2$ teaspoon salt
$^1/_8$ teaspoon pepper
$^1/_8$ teaspoon dried marjoram leaves
1 cup 2% reduced-fat milk
$^1/_2$ cup (2 ounces) shredded reduced-fat sharp Cheddar cheese
2 egg yolks
2 egg whites, beaten to stiff peaks

Place beans in greased 7 x 11-inch baking dish. Sauté onion in butter in small saucepan until tender, 1 to 2 minutes. Stir in flour, salt, pepper, and marjoram; cook 1 to 2 minutes, stirring constantly. Whisk in milk and heat to boiling; continue boiling, whisking, until thickened, 1 to 2 minutes. Pour sauce over beans.

Stir cheese into egg yolks; fold into egg whites. Spread egg mixture over sauce. Bake, uncovered, at 375 degrees until puffed and browned, about 20 minutes.

Makes 4 servings.

Nutritional Analysis per Serving

Vitamin A	268.3 RE	Vitamin D	1.1 µg
Thiamin (B-1)	0.1 mg	Vitamin E	0.9 mg
Riboflavin (B-2)	0.4 mg	Calcium	255.4 mg
Niacin	1.0 mg	Iron	1.7 mg
Vitamin B-6	0.1 mg	Phosphorus	146.3 mg
Vitamin B-12	0.5 µg	Magnesium	39.5 mg
Folate (total)	49.7 µg	Zinc	0.8 mg
Vitamin C	14.7 mg	Potassium	350.2 mg

Cheesy Potato Bake

PER SERVING: 270.8 CALORIES — 13.8 g PROTEIN — 45.0 g CARBOHYDRATE — 3.8 g FIBER —
4.4 g TOTAL FAT — 2.1 g SATURATED FAT — 6.2 mg CHOLESTEROL — 496.7 mg SODIUM

6 medium potatoes, peeled and thinly sliced
2 cups (4 ounces) shredded reduced-fat mozzarella cheese
1 package (2 ounces) white sauce mix
1 1/2 cups 2% reduced-fat milk
Salt and pepper, to taste
Paprika, as garnish

Alternate layers of potatoes and cheese in a greased 2-quart
baking dish (approximately 4 layers). Prepare white-sauce mix
according to package directions, using milk; season to taste with
salt and pepper. Pour sauce over potatoes; sprinkle with paprika.
Bake, covered, at 350 degrees, until potatoes are fork-tender,
45 to 60 minutes.

Makes 8 servings.

Nutritional Analysis per Serving

Vitamin A	86.2 RE	Vitamin D	0.5 µg
Thiamin (B-1)	0.2 mg	Vitamin E	0.2 mg
Riboflavin (B-2)	0.2 mg	Calcium	218.7 mg
Niacin	2.6 mg	Iron	2.1 mg
Vitamin B-6	0.6 mg	Phosphorus	147.2 mg
Vitamin B-12	0.2 µg	Magnesium	50.1 mg
Folate (total)	21.4 µg	Zinc	0.7 mg
Vitamin C	20.2 mg	Potassium	729.9 mg

Party Potatoes

PER SERVING: 322.2 CALORIES — 9.3 g PROTEIN — 54.7 g CARBOHYDRATE — 4.8 g FIBER —
7.1 g TOTAL FAT — 4.7 g SATURATED FAT — 23.3 mg CHOLESTEROL — 169.0 mg SODIUM

8 medium-size potatoes, peeled
1 package (8 ounces) reduced-fat cream cheese, softened
1 cup reduced-fat sour cream
Garlic salt and pepper, to taste

Cook potatoes and mash. Mix cream cheese and sour cream;
stir into potatoes, mixing well. Season to taste with garlic salt and
pepper. Spoon mixture into greased 1¹/₂-quart casserole. Bake,
uncovered, at 350 degrees until hot through, about 30 minutes.
Makes 8 servings.

Nutritional Analysis per Serving

Vitamin A	130.9 RE	Vitamin D	0.0 µg
Thiamin (B-1)	0.2 mg	Vitamin E	0.4 mg
Riboflavin (B-2)	0.2 mg	Calcium	115.6 mg
Niacin	3.4 mg	Iron	2.7 mg
Vitamin B-6	0.7 mg	Phosphorus	190.6 mg
Vitamin B-12	0.1 µg	Magnesium	54.5 mg
Folate (total)	26.0 µg	Zinc	0.6 mg
Vitamin C	26.1 mg	Potassium	963.1 mg

German Potatoes

PER SERVING: 293.2 CALORIES — 9.2 g PROTEIN — 53.4 g CARBOHYDRATE — 5.1 g FIBER —
5.2 g TOTAL FAT — 1.9 g SATURATED FAT — 78.1 mg CHOLESTEROL — 422.1 mg SODIUM

6 medium to large potatoes, peeled, shredded

1/2 cup finely chopped onion

2 eggs, beaten

1/2 cup whole milk

5 slices cooked bacon, very finely crumbled

3/4–1 teaspoon salt

1/2 teaspoon pepper

Mix all ingredients and spoon into greased 9 x 12-inch baking
dish. Bake, covered, at 375 degrees until potatoes are very tender,
45 to 60 minutes.

Makes 6 servings.

Nutritional Analysis per Serving

Vitamin A	38.2 RE	Vitamin D	0.4 µg
Thiamin (B-1)	0.3 mg	Vitamin E	0.3 mg
Riboflavin (B-2)	0.2 mg	Calcium	56.8 mg
Niacin	3.8 mg	Iron	3.2 mg
Vitamin B-6	0.8 mg	Phosphorus	186.1 mg
Vitamin B-12	0.3 µg	Magnesium	61.8 mg
Folate (total)	33.9 µg	Zinc	1.1 mg
Vitamin C	27.1 mg	Potassium	944.1 mg

Potato Casserole

PER SERVING: 378.4 CALORIES — 14.3 g PROTEIN — 61.1 g CARBOHYDRATE — 5.2 g FIBER —
8.6 g TOTAL FAT — 4.3 g SATURATED FAT — 127.2 mg CHOLESTEROL — 658.5 mg SODIUM

6 medium to large potatoes, peeled, quartered

1 cup reduced-fat sour cream

1 can (10³/₄ ounces) reduced-sodium, reduced-fat
cream of chicken soup (condensed)

¹/₂–³/₄ teaspoon curry powder

³/₄–1 teaspoon salt

¹/₂ teaspoon pepper

3 hard-cooked eggs, finely diced

¹/₂ cup fresh whole wheat bread crumbs

¹/₂ cup (2 ounces) shredded reduced-fat Cheddar cheese

Simmer potatoes in salted water until tender; cut into small
cubes. Mix sour cream, chicken soup, curry powder, salt, and
pepper in bowl. Layer the potatoes, eggs, and soup mixture in a
9 x 12-inch baking dish. Mix bread crumbs and cheese and sprinkle over the top. Bake, uncovered, at 350 degrees hot through,
about 30 minutes.

Makes 6 servings.

Nutritional Analysis per Serving

Vitamin A	210.5 RE	Vitamin D	0.4 µg
Thiamin (B-1)	0.2 mg	Vitamin E	0.4 mg
Riboflavin (B-2)	0.3 mg	Calcium	199.3 mg
Niacin	3.6 mg	Iron	3.3 mg
Vitamin B-6	0.7 mg	Phosphorus	221.5 mg
Vitamin B-12	0.4 µg	Magnesium	61.2 mg
Folate (total)	35.4 µg	Zinc	1.0 mg
Vitamin C	36.3 mg	Potassium	986.0 mg

Potato Pie

PER SERVING: 208.6 CALORIES — 16.5 g PROTEIN — 16.0 g CARBOHYDRATE — 1.4 g FIBER —
8.7 g TOTAL FAT — 3.8 g SATURATED FAT — 87.6 mg CHOLESTEROL — 608.8 mg SODIUM

1 carton (16 ounces) 2% creamed cottage cheese

2 cups mashed potatoes

$^1/_2$ cup reduced-fat sour cream

Salt and pepper, to taste

2 eggs

$^1/_4$–$^1/_2$ cup (1–2 ounces) shredded Parmesan cheese

Paprika, as garnish

Process cottage cheese in food processor or blender until smooth. Mix cottage cheese, mashed potatoes, and sour cream; season to taste with salt and pepper. Mix in eggs and Parmesan cheese and spoon into greased 1-quart casserole; sprinkle with paprika. Bake, covered, at 350 degrees until hot through, about 30 minutes; uncover and bake 10 minutes longer.

Makes 6 servings.

Nutritional Analysis per Serving

Vitamin A	106.7 RE	Vitamin D	0.3 µg
Thiamin (B-1)	0.1 mg	Vitamin E	0.5 mg
Riboflavin (B-2)	0.3 mg	Calcium	164.3 mg
Niacin	0.9 mg	Iron	0.6 mg
Vitamin B-6	0.2 mg	Phosphorus	229.4 mg
Vitamin B-12	0.8 µg	Magnesium	20.4 mg
Folate (total)	23.5 µg	Zinc	0.8 mg
Vitamin C	4.3 mg	Potassium	344.3 mg

Baked Hash Browns

PER SERVING: 251.1 CALORIES — 8.2 g PROTEIN — 34.1 g CARBOHYDRATE — 1.8 g FIBER —
9.7 g TOTAL FAT — 5.8 g SATURATED FAT — 24.6 mg CHOLESTEROL — 564.9 mg SODIUM

2 pounds frozen hash brown potatoes
1–2 cups (4–8 ounces) shredded reduced-fat Cheddar cheese
$1/2$ cup finely chopped onion
$1/2$ teaspoon salt
$1/4$ teaspoon pepper
1 can ($10^3/4$ ounces) reduced-sodium, reduced-fat
cream of chicken soup (condensed)
$1/4$ cup melted butter or margarine
1 cup finely crushed corn flakes

Combine potatoes, cheese, onion, salt, pepper, and chicken
soup in greased 2-quart casserole. Sprinkle combined butter and
cornflakes over potato mixture. Bake, uncovered, at 350 degrees
until hot through, 45 to 60 minutes.

Makes 8 servings.

Nutritional Analysis per Serving

Vitamin A	148.3 RE	Vitamin D	0.1 µg
Thiamin (B-1)	0.3 mg	Vitamin E	0.1 mg
Riboflavin (B-2)	0.2 mg	Calcium	140.5 mg
Niacin	2.3 mg	Iron	3.0 mg
Vitamin B-6	0.3 mg	Phosphorus	58.4 mg
Vitamin B-12	0.0 µg	Magnesium	13.8 mg
Folate (total)	15.8 µg	Zinc	0.3 mg
Vitamin C	15.2 mg	Potassium	356.7 mg

Cheese and Spinach Casserole

PER SERVING: 172.8 CALORIES — 16.4 g PROTEIN — 9.3 g CARBOHYDRATE — 2.2 g FIBER —
8.7 g TOTAL FAT — 4.9 g SATURATED FAT — 101.1 mg CHOLESTEROL — 625.7 mg SODIUM

2 packages (10 ounces each) frozen chopped spinach, thawed and well drained
1 carton (16 ounces) 1% reduced-fat creamed cottage cheese
3 eggs, beaten
1 1/2–2 cups (6–8 ounces) shredded reduced-fat American cheese
1 tablespoon melted butter or margarine
3 tablespoons flour
1/2 teaspoon salt
1/8 teaspoon pepper

Combine all ingredients, mixing well. Pour into greased
1 1/2-quart casserole. Bake, uncovered, at 350 degrees until set,
45 to 60 minutes.

Makes 8 servings.

Nutritional Analysis per Serving

Vitamin A	675.1 RE	Vitamin D	0.3 µg
Thiamin (B-1)	0.1 mg	Vitamin E	1.0 mg
Riboflavin (B-2)	0.3 mg	Calcium	335.9 mg
Niacin	0.6 mg	Iron	1.6 mg
Vitamin B-6	0.2 mg	Phosphorus	147.0 mg
Vitamin B-12	0.5 µg	Magnesium	54.3 mg
Folate (total)	96.7 µg	Zinc	0.9 mg
Vitamin C	8.7 mg	Potassium	286.7 mg

Spinach and Rice Casserole

PER SERVING: 161.4 CALORIES — 7.4 g PROTEIN — 15.5 g CARBOHYDRATE — 2.4 g FIBER — 8.6 g TOTAL FAT — 5.4 g SATURATED FAT — 21.4 mg CHOLESTEROL — 514.1 mg SODIUM

1 package (10 ounces) frozen chopped spinach, thawed, well drained
1 cup cooked rice
1 tablespoon finely grated onion
1/2–1 cup (2–4 ounces) shredded reduced-fat sharp Cheddar cheese
2–4 tablespoons butter or margarine
1/8 teaspoon ground nutmeg
1/2 teaspoon salt
1/8 teaspoon pepper

Combine all ingredients in medium bowl, mixing well; spoon into a greased 1-quart casserole. Bake, uncovered, at 375 degrees until hot through, about 30 minutes.

Makes 4 servings.

Nutritional Analysis per Serving

Vitamin A	668.0 RE	Vitamin D	0.1 µg
Thiamin (B-1)	0.1 mg	Vitamin E	0.8 mg
Riboflavin (B-2)	0.1 mg	Calcium	235.3 mg
Niacin	0.9 mg	Iron	1.6 mg
Vitamin B-6	0.1 mg	Phosphorus	53.8 mg
Vitamin B-12	0.0 µg	Magnesium	54.3 mg
Folate (total)	100.2 µg	Zinc	0.7 mg
Vitamin C	8.9 mg	Potassium	232.0 mg

Creamy Spinach–Onion Casserole

PER SERVING: 159.7 CALORIES — 10.5 g PROTEIN — 15.2 g CARBOHYDRATE — 4.3 g FIBER —
7.0 g TOTAL FAT — 4.0 g SATURATED FAT — 26.7 mg CHOLESTEROL — 581.9 mg SODIUM

3 packages (10 ounces each) chopped spinach, thawed, well drained
2 cups reduced-fat sour cream
1 envelope (1 ounce) dry onion-soup mix

Combine all ingredients and spoon into greased 1½-quart casserole. Bake, covered, at 350 degrees until hot through, about 30 minutes.

Makes 6 servings.

Nutritional Analysis per Serving

Vitamin A	1,262.8 RE	Vitamin D	.0 µg
Thiamin (B-1)	0.1 mg	Vitamin E	1.4 mg
Riboflavin (B-2)	0.4 mg	Calcium	367.0 mg
Niacin	0.6 mg	Iron	2.2 mg
Vitamin B-6	0.2 mg	Phosphorus	174.7 mg
Vitamin B-12	0.3 µg	Magnesium	97.8 mg
Folate (total)	153.1 µg	Zinc	1.0 mg
Vitamin C	17.4 mg	Potassium	609.1 mg

Cheesy Baked Spinach

PER SERVING: 131.1 CALORIES — 12.1 g PROTEIN — 9.0 g CARBOHYDRATE — 2.4 g FIBER —
6.2 g TOTAL FAT — 3.4 g SATURATED FAT — 65.5 mg CHOLESTEROL — 426.3 mg SODIUM

2 eggs, slightly beaten

2 cups 2% reduced-fat milk

$^1/_2$–1 teaspoon salt

$^1/_8$ teaspoon pepper

2 packages (10 ounces each) frozen chopped spinach, thawed, drained

$^2/_3$ cup fresh whole wheat bread crumbs

1$^1/_2$ cups (6 ounces) shredded reduced-fat brick cheese, divided

Paprika, as garnish

Combine eggs, milk, salt, and pepper in 2-quart casserole, mixing well. Stir in spinach, bread crumbs, and $^3/_4$ cup cheese. Sprinkle remaining $^3/_4$ cup cheese over casserole; sprinkle with paprika. Bake, uncovered, at 350 degrees until set, about 40 minutes.

Makes 8 servings.

Nutritional Analysis per Serving

Vitamin A	700.3 RE	Vitamin D	0.8 µg
Thiamin (B-1)	0.1 mg	Vitamin E	0.9 mg
Riboflavin (B-2)	0.3 mg	Calcium	373.6 mg
Niacin	0.5 mg	Iron	1.4 mg
Vitamin B-6	0.2 mg	Phosphorus	122.0 mg
Vitamin B-12	0.3 µg	Magnesium	62.2 mg
Folate (total)	86.7 µg	Zinc	0.9 mg
Vitamin C	9.3 mg	Potassium	334.1 mg

Garlic Spinach with Yogurt

PER SERVING: 43.3 CALORIES — 4.1 g PROTEIN — 6.5 g CARBOHYDRATE — 2.1 g FIBER —
0.7 g TOTAL FAT — 0.4 g SATURATED FAT — 2.1 mg CHOLESTEROL — 85.9 mg SODIUM

1 package (16 ounces) frozen chopped spinach, thawed, drained

1 carton (5 ounces) low-fat plain yogurt

1–2 cloves garlic, minced

Salt and pepper, to taste

Combine spinach, yogurt, and garlic in saucepan; cook over low heat until hot through. Season to taste with salt and pepper. Makes 4 servings.

Nutritional Analysis per Serving

Vitamin A	557.1 RE	Vitamin D	0.0 µg
Thiamin (B-1)	0.1 mg	Vitamin E	0.7 mg
Riboflavin (B-2)	0.2 mg	Calcium	169.7 mg
Niacin	0.3 mg	Iron	1.1 mg
Vitamin B-6	0.1 mg	Phosphorus	86.2 mg
Vitamin B-12	0.2 µg	Magnesium	55.1 mg
Folate (total)	80.5 µg	Zinc	0.8 mg
Vitamin C	9.2 mg	Potassium	297.1 mg

Herbed-Squash Casserole

PER SERVING: 92.3 CALORIES — 6.1 g PROTEIN — 7.4 g CARBOHYDRATE — 2.4 g FIBER —
5.0 g TOTAL FAT — 2.9 g SATURATED FAT — 13.0 mg CHOLESTEROL — 151.9 mg SODIUM

5 summer yellow squash, finely chopped

1 small onion, finely chopped

1–2 tablespoons butter or margarine

1 cup (4 ounces) shredded reduced-fat mozzarella or Cheddar cheese

3/4 teaspoon Italian seasoning

1/2 cup fresh whole wheat bread crumbs

Salt and pepper, to taste

Simmer squash and onion in saucepan until tender; drain and mash. Stir in butter, cheese, Italian seasoning, and bread crumbs, mixing well. Spoon into greased 1-quart casserole. Bake, covered, at 350 degrees until bread crumbs are browned, about 15 minutes. Season to taste with salt and pepper.

Makes 6 servings.

Nutritional Analysis per Serving

Vitamin A	98.8 RE	Vitamin D	0.0 µg
Thiamin (B-1)	0.1 mg	Vitamin E	0.2 mg
Riboflavin (B-2)	0.1 mg	Calcium	149.9 mg
Niacin	0.7 mg	Iron	0.6 mg
Vitamin B-6	0.1 mg	Phosphorus	147.2 mg
Vitamin B-12	0.2 µg	Magnesium	31.5 mg
Folate (total)	29.4 µg	Zinc	0.9 mg
Vitamin C	15.4 mg	Potassium	244.2 mg

Savory Garden Squash

PER SERVING: 70.3 CALORIES — 2.2 g PROTEIN — 8.0 g CARBOHYDRATE — 2.7 g FIBER —
3.3 g TOTAL FAT — 1.9 g SATURATED FAT — 8.2 mg CHOLESTEROL — 55.4 mg SODIUM

1 pound yellow or zucchini squash, chopped

1 small green bell pepper, chopped

1 small onion, chopped

$3/4$ cup peeled and chopped tomatoes

$1/2$ teaspoon dried savory leaves

$1/8$ teaspoon dried thyme leaves

1–2 tablespoons butter or margarine

Salt and pepper, to taste

Grated Parmesan cheese, as garnish

Simmer vegetables and herbs in water in saucepan until tender, 5 to 7 minutes; drain. Process in food processor or blender until smooth; stir in butter and season to taste with salt and pepper. Sprinkle with Parmesan cheese.

Makes 4 servings.

Nutritional Analysis per Serving

Vitamin A	69.0 RE	Vitamin D	0.1 µg
Thiamin (B-1)	0.0 mg	Vitamin E	0.4 mg
Riboflavin (B-2)	0.0 mg	Calcium	13.8 mg
Niacin	0.4 mg	Iron	0.5 mg
Vitamin B-6	0.1 mg	Phosphorus	21.5 mg
Vitamin B-12	0.0 µg	Magnesium	9.5 mg
Folate (total)	15.6 µg	Zinc	0.1 mg
Vitamin C	34.4 mg	Potassium	162.2 mg

Squash and Cornbread Stuffing Casserole

PER SERVING: 154.1 CALORIES — 5.9 g PROTEIN — 24.0 g CARBOHYDRATE — 5.0 g FIBER —
4.1 g TOTAL FAT — 2.0 g SATURATED FAT — 13.2 mg CHOLESTEROL — 357.3 mg SODIUM

2½ pounds summer yellow squash, chopped

1 medium onion, chopped

1 can (10¾ ounces) reduced-sodium, reduced-fat
cream of chicken soup (condensed)

1 cup reduced-fat sour cream

½ package (8 ounce-size) cornbread stuffing mix

Simmer squash and onion in water in saucepan until very
tender; drain and mash. Stir in remaining ingredients, mixing
well. Spoon into greased 2-quart casserole. Bake, covered, at
350 degrees until hot through, about 30 minutes.

Makes 8 servings.

Nutritional Analysis per Serving

Vitamin A	119.5 RE	Vitamin D	0.0 µg
Thiamin (B-1)	0.2 mg	Vitamin E	0.2 mg
Riboflavin (B-2)	0.2 mg	Calcium	100.7 mg
Niacin	1.5 mg	Iron	1.1 mg
Vitamin B-6	0.2 mg	Phosphorus	105.2 mg
Vitamin B-12	0.1 µg	Magnesium	38.6 mg
Folate (total)	48.1 µg	Zinc	0.5 mg
Vitamin C	25.8 mg	Potassium	369.3 mg

Sweet Potato Purée

PER SERVING: 222.2 CALORIES — 2.9 g PROTEIN — 38.8 g CARBOHYDRATE — 5.6 g FIBER —
6.8 g TOTAL FAT — 4.0 g SATURATED FAT — 17.5 mg CHOLESTEROL — 83.4 mg SODIUM

2 sweet potatoes, peeled, cooked, warm

1–2 tablespoons butter or margarine

1–2 tablespoons whole milk

1–2 tablespoons orange juice concentrate

Finely grated rind of 1/2 orange

1/2 teaspoon ground cinnamon

Salt and pepper, to taste

Mash sweet potatoes, adding butter, milk, orange juice concentrate, orange rind, and cinnamon; season to taste with salt and pepper.

Makes 2 servings.

Nutritional Analysis per Serving

Vitamin A	2,674.4 RE	Vitamin D	0.2 µg
Thiamin (B-1)	0.1 mg	Vitamin E	0.5 mg
Riboflavin (B-2)	0.2 mg	Calcium	68.7 mg
Niacin	1.1 mg	Iron	1.1 mg
Vitamin B-6	0.4 mg	Phosphorus	53.1 mg
Vitamin B-12	0.0 µg	Magnesium	20.1 mg
Folate (total)	36.3 µg	Zinc	0.5 mg
Vitamin C	58.3 mg	Potassium	366.9 mg

Steamed Sweet Potatoes and Parsnips

PER SERVING: 158.7 CALORIES — 2.1 g PROTEIN — 30.9 g CARBOHYDRATE — 5.3 g FIBER —
3.5 g TOTAL FAT — 2.0 g SATURATED FAT — 8.2 mg CHOLESTEROL — 47.7 mg SODIUM

1 1/2 pounds sweet potatoes, peeled and thinly sliced
1 pound parsnips, peeled and thinly sliced
2–4 tablespoons butter or margarine
Ground cinnamon, to taste
Ground nutmeg, to taste
Salt and pepper, to taste

Cook sweet potatoes and parsnips in 1/2-inch simmering water until very tender, 2 to 3 minutes. Drain well. Season to taste with butter, cinnamon, nutmeg, salt, and pepper.

Makes 8 servings.

Nutritional Analysis per Serving

Vitamin A	1,734.3 RE	Vitamin D	0.1 µg
Thiamin (B-1)	0.1 mg	Vitamin E	0.3 mg
Riboflavin (B-2)	0.2 mg	Calcium	40.0 mg
Niacin	1.0 mg	Iron	0.8 mg
Vitamin B-6	0.3 mg	Phosphorus	64.9 mg
Vitamin B-12	0.0 µg	Magnesium	25.0 mg
Folate (total)	50.0 µg	Zinc	0.6 mg
Vitamin C	28.9 mg	Potassium	387.1 mg

Southern Sweet Potatoes

PER SERVING: 299.2 CALORIES — 4.3 g PROTEIN — 58.3 g CARBOHYDRATE — 3.9 g FIBER —
6.3 g TOTAL FAT — 3.3 g SATURATED FAT — 82.9 mg CHOLESTEROL — 133.8 mg SODIUM

2 cans (16 ounces each) sweet potatoes, undrained
2 eggs, lightly beaten
2 tablespoons melted butter or margarine
$1/2$ cup honey
3 tablespoons flour
3 tablespoons whole milk

Mash sweet potatoes and mix in eggs; spoon into greased 1-quart casserole. Combine butter, honey, flour, and milk; pour over sweet potatoes. Bake, uncovered, at 350 degrees until hot through, about 30 minutes.

Makes 6 servings.

Nutritional Analysis per Serving

Vitamin A	936.7 RE	Vitamin D	0.4 µg
Thiamin (B-1)	0.1 mg	Vitamin E	0.6 mg
Riboflavin (B-2)	0.2 mg	Calcium	43.4 mg
Niacin	1.0 mg	Iron	1.8 mg
Vitamin B-6	0.1 mg	Phosphorus	84.1 mg
Vitamin B-12	0.2 µg	Magnesium	23.8 mg
Folate (total)	25.5 µg	Zinc	0.6 mg
Vitamin C	16.1 mg	Potassium	331.5 mg

Sweet Potato and Apple Casserole

PER SERVING: 329.6 CALORIES — 3.6 g PROTEIN — 73.2 g CARBOHYDRATE — 4.3 g FIBER —
3.7 g TOTAL FAT — 2.0 g SATURATED FAT — 8.2 mg CHOLESTEROL — 59.7 mg SODIUM

5 cups mashed cooked sweet potatoes

1 1/2 cups unsweetened applesauce

1/2 cup honey

2 tablespoons orange juice

2 tablespoons butter or margarine

Ground cinnamon

Spoon sweet potatoes into greased 2-quart casserole; spoon applesauce over the potatoes. Combine honey and orange juice and drizzle over top. Dot with butter and sprinkle generously with cinnamon. Bake, uncovered, at 350 degrees until hot through, about 30 minutes.

Makes 8 servings.

Nutritional Analysis per Serving

Vitamin A	3,560.9 RE	Vitamin D	0.1 µg
Thiamin (B-1)	0.1 mg	Vitamin E	0.6 mg
Riboflavin (B-2)	0.3 mg	Calcium	47.4 mg
Niacin	1.5 mg	Iron	1.3 mg
Vitamin B-6	0.5 mg	Phosphorus	61.5 mg
Vitamin B-12	0.0 µg	Magnesium	23.0 mg
Folate (total)	24.9 µg	Zinc	0.6 mg
Vitamin C	38.0 mg	Potassium	435.0 mg

Wild Rice–Tomato Casserole

PER SERVING: 325.1 CALORIES — 16.9 g PROTEIN — 49.0 g CARBOHYDRATE — 4.6 g FIBER —
8.5 g TOTAL FAT — 3.8 g SATURATED FAT — 15.0 mg CHOLESTEROL — 506.6 mg SODIUM

$^1/_2$ pound mushrooms, finely chopped

$^1/_2$ cup minced onion

$^1/_4$ cup finely chopped green bell pepper

$^1/_4$ cup finely chopped red bell pepper

1–2 tablespoons olive oil

1 can (19-ounces) herb-seasoned tomatoes, undrained, finely chopped

2 cups (8 ounces) shredded mozzarella cheese, grated

1 package (16 ounces) wild rice, cooked, warm

Salt and pepper, to taste

Sauté mushrooms, onion, and peppers in oil in a large skillet. Add tomatoes, cheese, and wild rice, mixing well; season to taste with salt and pepper. Spoon mixture into greased 3-quart casserole. Bake, covered, at 350 degrees until hot through, about 30 minutes.

Makes 8 servings.

Nutritional Analysis per Serving

Vitamin A	129.0 RE	Vitamin D	0.5 µg
Thiamin (B-1)	0.1 mg	Vitamin E	0.8 mg
Riboflavin (B-2)	0.3 mg	Calcium	237.7 mg
Niacin	4.8 mg	Iron	1.8 mg
Vitamin B-6	0.3 mg	Phosphorus	255.5 mg
Vitamin B-12	0.0 µg	Magnesium	100.1 mg
Folate (total)	39.7 µg	Zinc	3.4 mg
Vitamin C	24.1 mg	Potassium	342.9 mg

Zucchini Au Gratin

PER SERVING: 94.6 CALORIES — 5.7 g PROTEIN — 9.2 g CARBOHYDRATE — 3.0 g FIBER —
4.8 g TOTAL FAT — 1.2 g SATURATED FAT — 4.3 mg CHOLESTEROL — 454.1 mg SODIUM

4 medium zucchini

1 small onion, minced

1 clove garlic, minced

1–2 tablespoons vegetable oil

$^1/_2$ teaspoon salt

$^1/_4$ teaspoon pepper

2 tablespoons grated Parmesan cheese

$^1/_4$ cup tomato sauce

$^1/_4$–$^1/_2$ cup (1–2 ounces) shredded reduced-fat Swiss cheese

Sauté zucchini, onion, and garlic in oil in medium skillet until tender, about 5 minutes. Stir in salt, pepper, and Parmesan cheese; transfer to greased 1-quart casserole. Drizzle with tomato sauce and sprinkle with Swiss cheese. Bake, uncovered, at 350 degrees, until cheese melts, about 15 minutes.

Makes 4 servings.

Nutritional Analysis per Serving

Vitamin A	90.4 RE	Vitamin D	0.0 µg
Thiamin (B-1)	0.2 mg	Vitamin E	1.2 mg
Riboflavin (B-2)	0.1 mg	Calcium	137.0 mg
Niacin	1.0 mg	Iron	1.1 mg
Vitamin B-6	0.2 mg	Phosphorus	136.7 mg
Vitamin B-12	0.1 µg	Magnesium	52.2 mg
Folate (total)	48.9 µg	Zinc	0.8 mg
Vitamin C	21.2 mg	Potassium	589.2 mg

Zucchini Mexicali

PER SERVING: 182.2 CALORIES — 12.8 g PROTEIN — 10.5 g CARBOHYDRATE — 2.4 g FIBER —
10.7 g TOTAL FAT — 5.9 g SATURATED FAT — 131.0 mg CHOLESTEROL — 593.6 mg SODIUM

2 pounds zucchini, cubed, cooked

$1/2$ cup 1% low-fat milk

4 eggs, beaten

3 tablespoons flour

1 teaspoon baking powder

$1/2$ teaspoon ground cumin

$1/2$ teaspoon salt

$1/4$ teaspoon pepper

2 cups (8 ounces) shredded reduced-fat Monterey Jack cheese

$1/4$ cup finely chopped parsley

1 can (4-ounces) mild or hot green chilies, finely chopped

1 cup fresh whole wheat bread crumbs

1–2 tablespoons melted butter or margarine

Spoon zucchini into greased 2-quart casserole. Beat milk and eggs in medium bowl until well blended; beat in flour, baking powder, cumin, salt, and pepper. Mix in cheese, parsley, and chilies; spoon over zucchini in casserole. Toss bread crumbs and butter; sprinkle over casserole. Bake at 325 degrees until puffed and browned, 30 to 40 minutes.

Makes 8 servings.

Nutritional Analysis per Serving

Vitamin A	237.9 RE	Vitamin D	0.5 µg
Thiamin (B-1)	0.1 mg	Vitamin E	0.5 mg
Riboflavin (B-2)	0.3 mg	Calcium	308.6 mg
Niacin	0.9 mg	Iron	1.3 mg
Vitamin B-6	0.1 mg	Phosphorus	274.4 mg
Vitamin B-12	0.6 µg	Magnesium	44.7 mg
Folate (total)	43.0 µg	Zinc	2.2 mg
Vitamin C	14.2 mg	Potassium	418.1 mg

Braised Red Cabbage and Apples

PER SERVING: 174.4 CALORIES — 3.3 g PROTEIN — 39.9 g CARBOHYDRATE — 5.8 g FIBER —
2.6 g TOTAL FAT — 1.3 g SATURATED FAT — 5.5 mg CHOLESTEROL — 56.7 mg SODIUM

1 small red cabbage, finely chopped

2 apples, grated

$1/4$ cup finely chopped onion

$1/2$ cup cider vinegar

$1/2$ cup water

$1/2$ cup honey

1 teaspoon crushed caraway seeds

1 tablespoon butter or margarine

Salt and pepper, to taste

Heat all ingredients, except salt and pepper, to boiling in large saucepan; reduce heat and simmer, covered, until cabbage is very tender, 30 to 40 minutes, adding small amount of water, if needed. Season to taste with salt and pepper.

Makes 6 servings.

Nutritional Analysis per Serving

Vitamin A	37.4 RE	Vitamin D	0.0 µg
Thiamin (B-1)	0.1 mg	Vitamin E	0.2 mg
Riboflavin (B-2)	0.1 mg	Calcium	96.9 mg
Niacin	0.6 mg	Iron	1.0 mg
Vitamin B-6	0.3 mg	Phosphorus	10.9 mg
Vitamin B-12	0.0 µg	Magnesium	40.2 mg
Folate (total)	3.4 µg	Zinc	0.4 mg
Vitamin C	97.9 mg	Potassium	533.8 mg

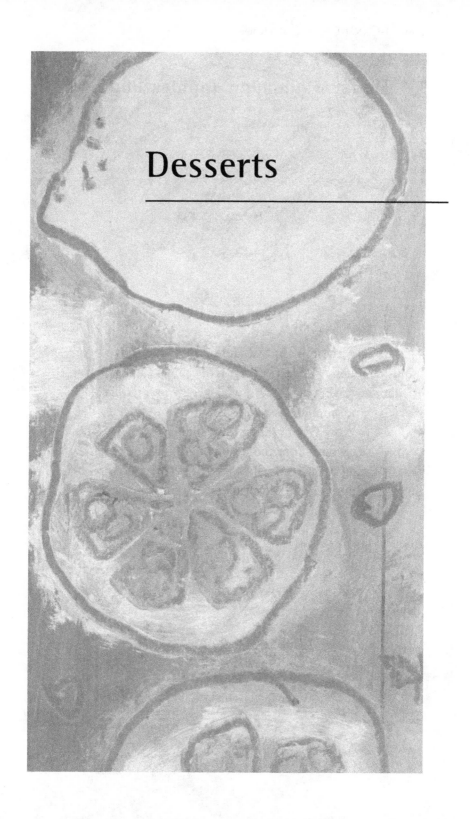

Desserts

Honey-Cinnamon Tapioca Pudding

PER SERVING: 214.0 CALORIES — 7.2 g PROTEIN — 31.6 g CARBOHYDRATE — 0.0 g FIBER —
6.6 g TOTAL FAT — 3.3 g SATURATED FAT — 123.4 mg CHOLESTEROL — 164.5 mg SODIUM

2 tablespoons minute tapioca

2 cups whole milk

1/4 cup honey

1/8 teaspoon salt

2 egg yolks

2–3 teaspoons vanilla

2 egg whites

1 tablespoon sugar

Ground cinnamon, as garnish

Mix tapioca, milk, honey, and salt in medium saucepan; let stand 5 minutes. Heat to boiling; reduce heat to low. Whisk about 1/2 cup mixture into egg yolks; whisk egg yolk mixture back into saucepan and simmer, stirring constantly, until thickened, 8 to 10 minutes. Remove from heat; stir in vanilla. Cool 5 minutes.

Beat egg whites in medium bowl until foamy; beat to soft peaks, adding sugar gradually. Fold egg whites into tapioca. Refrigerate and serve cold; sprinkle with cinnamon.

Makes 4 servings.

Nutritional Analysis per Serving

Vitamin A	86.3 RE	Vitamin D	1.5 µg
Thiamin (B-1)	0.1 mg	Vitamin E	0.4 mg
Riboflavin (B-2)	0.3 mg	Calcium	159.1 mg
Niacin	0.2 mg	Iron	0.5 mg
Vitamin B-6	0.1 mg	Phosphorus	157.2 mg
Vitamin B-12	0.7 µg	Magnesium	19.1 mg
Folate (total)	19.1 µg	Zinc	0.8 mg
Vitamin C	1.2 mg	Potassium	231.2 mg

Orange Pudding Cake

PER SERVING: 315.3 CALORIES — 9.5 g PROTEIN — 42.6 g CARBOHYDRATE — 0.6 g FIBER —
12.5 g TOTAL FAT — 6.1 g SATURATED FAT — 234.0 mg CHOLESTEROL — 155.9 mg SODIUM

$^1/_2$ cup honey

2 tablespoons butter or margarine

1$^1/_2$ tablespoons grated orange rind

4 egg yolks

$^1/_4$ cup all-purpose flour

1 cup 2% reduced-fat milk

$^1/_2$ cup orange juice

4 egg whites

$^1/_4$ cup sugar*

Mix honey, butter, and orange rind. Add egg yolks one at a time, beating well after each addition. Mix in flour, milk, and orange juice. Beat egg whites in large bowl until foamy; beat to stiff peaks, adding sugar gradually. Fold egg whites into batter.

Pour batter into greased 1$^1/_2$-quart casserole. Bake at 350 degrees until cake is browned and springs back when touched, about 30 minutes.

Makes 4 servings.

*Can replace with 8 packets of Equal.

Nutritional Analysis per Serving

Vitamin A	195.4 RE	Vitamin D	1.3 µg
Thiamin (B-1)	0.1 mg	Vitamin E	0.7 mg
Riboflavin (B-2)	0.4 mg	Calcium	110.6 mg
Niacin	0.7 mg	Iron	1.2 mg
Vitamin B-6	0.1 mg	Phosphorus	160.3 mg
Vitamin B-12	0.8 µg	Magnesium	19.9 mg
Folate (total)	50.9 µg	Zinc	0.9 mg
Vitamin C	19.3 mg	Potassium	245.5 mg

Chocolate Velvet Pudding

PER SERVING: 315.4 CALORIES — 3.6 g PROTEIN — 45.4 g CARBOHYDRATE — 1.6 g FIBER —
12.5 g TOTAL FAT — 9.7 g SATURATED FAT — 4.9 mg CHOLESTEROL — 385.0 mg SODIUM

1 package (3½ ounces) instant chocolate pudding and pie filling
1 cup 2% reduced-fat milk
2 ounces semi-sweet baking chocolate, melted
1 carton (8 ounces) frozen reduced-fat, nondairy whipped topping, thawed

Prepare pudding according to package directions, using milk.
Gradually mix in chocolate. Fold in whipped topping. Spoon into
dessert glasses and chill, or freeze until firm, about 4 hours.

Makes 4 servings.

Nutritional Analysis per Serving

Vitamin A	34.8 RE	Vitamin D	0.6 µg
Thiamin (B-1)	0 mg	Vitamin E	0.2 mg
Riboflavin (B-2)	0.1 mg	Calcium	78.4 mg
Niacin	0.2 mg	Iron	1.3 mg
Vitamin B-6	0 mg	Phosphorus	331.1 mg
Vitamin B-12	0.2 µg	Magnesium	39.9 mg
Folate (total)	4.4 µg	Zinc	0.9 mg
Vitamin C	0.6 mg	Potassium	223.4 mg

Honey-Scented Vanilla Pudding

PER SERVING: 164.8 CALORIES — 5.7 g PROTEIN — 27.2 g CARBOHYDRATE — 0.1 g FIBER —
3.6 g TOTAL FAT — 1.8 g SATURATED FAT — 62.9 mg CHOLESTEROL — 78.1 mg SODIUM

$1/4$ cup honey

2 tablespoons cornstarch

2 cups 2% reduced-fat milk

1 egg, beaten

2–3 teaspoons vanilla

Mix honey and cornstarch in medium saucepan; whisk in milk and heat to boiling. Whisk about $1/2$ cup milk mixture into egg; whisk egg mixture back into saucepan. Reduce heat and simmer rapidly, whisking constantly, until thickened. Stir in vanilla. Serve warm, or refrigerate and serve cold.

Makes 4 servings.

Nutritional Analysis per Serving

Vitamin A	93.4 RE	Vitamin D	1.4 µg
Thiamin (B-1)	0.1 mg	Vitamin E	0.2 mg
Riboflavin (B-2)	0.3 mg	Calcium	156.5 mg
Niacin	0.1 mg	Iron	0.4 mg
Vitamin B-6	0.1 mg	Phosphorus	139.6 mg
Vitamin B-12	0.6 µg	Magnesium	19.1 mg
Folate (total)	12.4 µg	Zinc	0.7 mg
Vitamin C	1.3 mg	Potassium	217.2 mg

Creamy Banana Pudding

PER SERVING: 206.7 CALORIES — 6.4 g PROTEIN — 33.2 g CARBOHYDRATE — 1.0 g FIBER —
5.9 g TOTAL FAT — 2.6 g SATURATED FAT — 151.5 mg CHOLESTEROL — 115.7 mg SODIUM

3 cups 2% reduced-fat milk
$^1/_3$ cup honey
1 tablespoon cornstarch
4 egg yolks, beaten
2 large ripe bananas, mashed
$1^1/_2$ teaspoons vanilla extract
$^1/_8$ teaspoon salt

Mix milk, honey, and cornstarch in large saucepan; heat to boiling, stirring frequently. Whisk about 1 cup milk mixture into egg yolks; whisk egg yolks back into saucepan. Reduce heat and simmer, whisking constantly, until thickened. Remove from heat and stir in bananas, vanilla, and salt. Serve warm, or refrigerate and serve chilled.

Makes 6 servings.

Nutritional Analysis per Serving

Vitamin A	137.3 RE	Vitamin D	1.6 µg
Thiamin (B-1)	0.1 mg	Vitamin E	0.5 mg
Riboflavin (B-2)	0.3 mg	Calcium	167.7 mg
Niacin	0.3 mg	Iron	0.7 mg
Vitamin B-6	0.3 mg	Phosphorus	178.9 mg
Vitamin B-12	0.8 µg	Magnesium	30.1 mg
Folate (total)	30.1 µg	Zinc	0.9 mg
Vitamin C	4.9 mg	Potassium	365.4 mg

Cherry Angel Trifle

PER SERVING: 303.8 CALORIES — 6.3 g PROTEIN — 61.1 g CARBOHYDRATE — 1.1 g FIBER — 3.8 g TOTAL FAT — 2.1 g SATURATED FAT — 13.7 mg CHOLESTEROL — 553.5 mg SODIUM

8 cups angel food cake, cut into small cubes, divided
1 can (21 ounces) cherry pie filling, divided
1 package (3.8 ounces) instant vanilla pudding
1½ cups 2% reduced-fat milk
1 cup reduced-fat sour cream

Place half of the cake cubes into a 9 x 13 x 2-inch baking pan. Reserve ⅓ cup cherry pie filling. Spoon remaining pie filling over cake cubes. Top with remaining cake cubes. Combine pudding mix, milk, and sour cream in mixer bowl; beat until smooth. Mix in reserved ⅓ cup pie filling and spoon over top of cake. Cover and refrigerate until chilled.

Makes 8 servings.

Nutritional Analysis per Serving

Vitamin A	101.7 RE	Vitamin D	0.5 µg
Thiamin (B-1)	0.1 mg	Vitamin E	0.0 mg
Riboflavin (B-2)	0.4 mg	Calcium	185.0 mg
Niacin	0.5 mg	Iron	0.4 mg
Vitamin B-6	0.1 mg	Phosphorus	195.7 mg
Vitamin B-12	0.3 µg	Magnesium	16.8 mg
Folate (total)	20.1 µg	Zinc	0.3 mg
Vitamin C	3.2 mg	Potassium	259.6 mg

Chocolate Bread Pudding

PER SERVING: 316.9 CALORIES — 9.7 g PROTEIN — 53.4 g CARBOHYDRATE — 1.1 g FIBER —
8.6 g TOTAL FAT — 4.0 g SATURATED FAT — 150.8 mg CHOLESTEROL — 180.9 mg SODIUM

2 eggs
2³/₄ cups 2% reduced-fat milk
²/₃ cup honey
1 ounce unsweetened baking chocolate, melted
1 teaspoon vanilla
2 cups fresh white coarse bread crumbs
2 egg whites
¹/₄ cup sugar*

Mix eggs, milk, honey, melted chocolate, and vanilla in large bowl; mix in bread crumbs and pour into greased 1¹/₂-quart casserole. Bake, uncovered, at 350 degrees until set, 30 to 45 minutes.

Beat egg whites in medium bowl until foamy; beat to stiff peaks, adding sugar gradually. Spoon over bread pudding and continue baking until lightly browned, about 10 minutes.

Makes 6 servings.

*Can substitute 8 packets of Equal.

Nutritional Analysis per Serving

Vitamin A	127.9 RE	Vitamin D	1.6 µg
Thiamin (B-1)	0.1 mg	Vitamin E	0.5 mg
Riboflavin (B-2)	0.4 mg	Calcium	174.9 mg
Niacin	0.8 mg	Iron	1.5 mg
Vitamin B-6	0.1 mg	Phosphorus	201.1 mg
Vitamin B-12	0.7 µg	Magnesium	38.1 mg
Folate (total)	36.6 µg	Zinc	1.2 mg
Vitamin C	1.3 mg	Potassium	290.5 mg

Bread and Butter Pudding

PER SERVING: 345.5 CALORIES — 9.4 g PROTEIN — 43.2 g CARBOHYDRATE — 0.8 g FIBER —
15.6 g TOTAL FAT — 8.0 g SATURATED FAT — 192.1 mg CHOLESTEROL — 343.7 mg SODIUM

10 slices white bread, crusts removed

4 tablespoons butter or margarine, softened

4 eggs

2 egg yolks

²/₃ cup honey

1 teaspoon vanilla

¹/₈ teaspoon salt

2 cups 2% reduced-fat milk

1 cup half-and-half

Butter bread slices lightly on top sides. Layer bread, buttered sides up, in generously buttered 9 x 13-inch baking pan, cutting slices to fit, if necessary.

Beat eggs, yolks, honey, vanilla, and salt in large bowl. Heat milk and half-and-half to simmering in medium saucepan; whisk into egg mixture. Pour over bread in baking pan. Let stand for 20 minutes.

Set baking dish in a larger baking pan; pour 1-inch hot water into pan. Bake at 325 degrees until browned, about 1 hour.

Place under hot broiler for a few minutes to glaze, watching carefully to make sure it does not burn.

Makes 8 servings.

Nutritional Analysis per Serving

Vitamin A	195.4 RE	Vitamin D	1.2 µg
Thiamin (B-1)	0.2 mg	Vitamin E	0.7 mg
Riboflavin (B-2)	0.4 mg	Calcium	161.2 mg
Niacin	1.4 mg	Iron	1.6 mg
Vitamin B-6	0.1 mg	Phosphorus	183.5 mg
Vitamin B-12	0.7 µg	Magnesium	22.7 mg
Folate (total)	52.2 µg	Zinc	1.1 mg
Vitamin C	1.0 mg	Potassium	221.6 mg

Nectarine–Orange Ice

PER SERVING: 114.3 CALORIES — 0.9 g PROTEIN — 28.4 g CARBOHYDRATE — 1.2 g FIBER —
0.4 g TOTAL FAT — 0.0 g SATURATED FAT — 0.0 mg CHOLESTEROL — 0.6 mg SODIUM

3 cups cubed, peeled, pitted nectarines (about 6)
1 cup fresh orange juice
$^1/_2$ cup sugar*

Process all ingredients in food processor or blender until
smooth. Freeze mixture in ice cream machine according to manufacturer's directions. Or, pour mixture into 11 x 7-inch baking
pan and freeze until slushy. Place in bowl and beat to break up ice
crystals; return to pan and freeze until firm. To serve, let stand at
room temperature until soft enough to scoop, about 10 minutes.

Makes 6 servings.

*Can substitute 12 packets of Equal, but keep in mind that the texture becomes significantly
harder/icelike and scooping becomes impossible when Equal is used.

Nutritional Analysis per Serving

Vitamin A	59.3 RE	Vitamin D	0.0 µg
Thiamin (B-1)	0.0 mg	Vitamin E	0.7 mg
Riboflavin (B-2)	0.0 mg	Calcium	8.2 mg
Niacin	0.8 mg	Iron	0.2 mg
Vitamin B-6	0.0 mg	Phosphorus	18.4 mg
Vitamin B-12	0.0 µg	Magnesium	10.1 mg
Folate (total)	15.2 µg	Zinc	0.1 mg
Vitamin C	24.4 mg	Potassium	229.3 mg

Lime–Banana Ice

PER SERVING: 163.1 CALORIES — 1.5 g PROTEIN — 43.2 g CARBOHYDRATE — 3.2 g FIBER —
0.6 g TOTAL FAT — 0.2 g SATURATED FAT — 0.0 mg CHOLESTEROL — 2.3 mg SODIUM

2 cups water
1 cup lime juice
1/4 cup honey
2 tablespoons finely grated lime rind
4 dashes ground nutmeg
6 ripe large bananas, peeled

Process all ingredients in food processor or blender until
smooth. Freeze mixture in ice cream machine according to manufacturer's directions. Or, pour into 9 x 13-inch baking pan and
freeze until slushy. Place in bowl; beat to break up ice crystals.
Return to pan and freeze until firm. To serve, remove from freezer
and let stand until soft enough to scrape up ice crystals with a
spoon, about 10 minutes.

Makes 6 serving.

Nutritional Analysis per Serving

Vitamin A	10.0 RE	Vitamin D	0.0 µg
Thiamin (B-1)	0.1 mg	Vitamin E	0.4 mg
Riboflavin (B-2)	0.1 mg	Calcium	14.3 mg
Niacin	0.7 mg	Iron	0.5 mg
Vitamin B-6	0.7 mg	Phosphorus	27.3 mg
Vitamin B-12	0.0 µg	Magnesium	37.3 mg
Folate (total)	26.2 µg	Zinc	0.2 mg
Vitamin C	25.4 mg	Potassium	522.5 mg

Plum and Strawberry Ice

PER SERVING: 209.0 CALORIES — 1.8 g PROTEIN — 51.5 g CARBOHYDRATE — 4.2 g FIBER —
1.3 g TOTAL FAT — 0.1 g SATURATED FAT — 0 mg CHOLESTEROL — 1.0 mg SODIUM

1 1/2 pounds fresh plums, halved, pitted
1 pint strawberries, hulled
1/2 cup water
1 tablespoon lemon juice
1/2 cup sugar*

Heat all ingredients to boiling in medium saucepan; reduce heat and simmer, covered, 5 minutes or until plums are tender. Cool. Process mixture in a food processor or blender until smooth. Cool.

Freeze mixture in ice cream machine according to manufacturer's directions. Or, pour into a 7 x 11-inch baking pan and freeze until slushy. Place in bowl, beat to break up ice crystals. Return to pan and freeze until firm. To serve, remove from freezer and let stand until soft enough to scrape up ice crystals with a spoon, about 10 minutes.

Makes 4 servings.

*Can substitute 2 packets of Equal

Nutritional Analysis per Serving

Vitamin A	56.7 RE	Vitamin D	0.0 μg
Thiamin (B-1)	0.1 mg	Vitamin E	1.1 mg
Riboflavin (B-2)	0.2 mg	Calcium	17.4 mg
Niacin	1.0 mg	Iron	0.5 mg
Vitamin B-6	0.2 mg	Phosphorus	31.4 mg
Vitamin B-12	0.0 μg	Magnesium	19.3 mg
Folate (total)	16.9 μg	Zinc	0.3 mg
Vitamin C	58.7 mg	Potassium	417.3 mg

Fruit Sherbet

PER SERVING: 125.6 CALORIES — 6.8 g PROTEIN — 21.4 g CARBOHYDRATE — 0.7 g FIBER —
2.3 g TOTAL FAT — 1.3 g SATURATED FAT — 8.5 mg CHOLESTEROL — 75.6 mg SODIUM

3 cups peeled, seeded ripe fruit (any kind)
2 envelopes unflavored gelatin
1/4 cup honey
1 1/2 cups whole milk
1/2 cup no-cholesterol real egg product, optional**

Process all ingredients in food processor or blender until
smooth. Freeze in ice cream machine according to manufacturer's
directions. Or, pour mixture into 11 x 7-inch baking pan and
freeze until slushy. Place in bowl and beat to break up ice crystals;
return to pan and freeze until firm. To serve, remove from freezer
and let stand at room temperature until soft enough to scoop,
about 10 minutes.

Makes 6 servings.

**Nutritional computations include information on no cholesterol real-egg product

Nutritional Analysis per Serving

Vitamin A	296.5 RE	Vitamin D	0.7 µg
Thiamin (B-1)	0.1 mg	Vitamin E	0.4 mg
Riboflavin (B-2)	0.5 mg	Calcium	90.2 mg
Niacin	0.6 mg	Iron	0.6 mg
Vitamin B-6	0.1 mg	Phosphorus	85.1 mg
Vitamin B-12	0.4 µg	Magnesium	18.9 mg
Folate (total)	28.3 µg	Zinc	0.6 mg
Vitamin C	34.4 mg	Potassium	375.9 mg

Spiced Fruit Compote

PER SERVING: 179.7 CALORIES — 0.9 g PROTEIN — 42.6 g CARBOHYDRATE — 2.5 g FIBER —
2.2 g TOTAL FAT — 1.3 g SATURATED FAT — 5.5 mg CHOLESTEROL — 35.1 mg SODIUM

2 cans (15¼ ounces) crushed pineapple, drained
1 can (16 ounces) pear halves, drained, finely chopped
1 can (16 ounces) peach halves, drained, finely chopped
1 can (16 ounces) apricot halves, drained, finely chopped
1 jar (6 ounces) maraschino cherries, drained, finely chopped
¹/₂ cup honey
¹/₂ teaspoon ground cloves
¹/₂ teaspoon ground allspice
¹/₄ teaspoon ground cinnamon
2–4 tablespoons melted butter or margarine

Combine fruit in a baking dish. Mix remaining ingredients
and pour over fruit; dot with butter. Bake, covered, at 350 degrees
until hot, about 30 minutes.

Makes 12 servings.

Nutritional Analysis per Serving

Vitamin A	100.1 RE	Vitamin D	0.0 µg
Thiamin (B-1)	0.1 mg	Vitamin E	1.0 mg
Riboflavin (B-2)	0.0 mg	Calcium	22.1 mg
Niacin	0.6 mg	Iron	0.7 mg
Vitamin B-6	0.1 mg	Phosphorus	21.5 mg
Vitamin B-12	0.0 µg	Magnesium	17.5 mg
Folate (total)	6.0 µg	Zinc	0.2 mg
Vitamin C	10.6 mg	Potassium	265.8 mg

Rich Coffee Crème

PER SERVING: 229.3 CALORIES — 7.9 g PROTEIN — 34.7 g CARBOHYDRATE — 0.4 g FIBER —
6.3 g TOTAL FAT — 2.7 g SATURATED FAT — 169.2 mg CHOLESTEROL — 67.2 mg SODIUM

2 cups 2% reduced-fat milk, divided
2–3 teaspoons instant coffee crystals
3 egg yolks
$^1/_3$ cup sugar*
$^1/_2$ cup all-purpose flour
$^1/_2$ teaspoon cornstarch
$^1/_2$ teaspoon vanilla extract

Heat milk and instant coffee to simmering in saucepan, stirring to dissolve coffee. Mix egg yolks, sugar, flour, and cornstarch in bowl. Whisk about half the milk and coffee mixture into yolk mixture; whisk yolk mixture into remaining milk in saucepan. Cook over low heat, whisking constantly, until thickened. Stir in vanilla extract and cool. Refrigerate until chilled.

Makes 4 servings.

*Can substitute 10 packets of Equal

Nutritional Analysis per Serving

Vitamin A	142.2 RE	Vitamin D	1.7 µg
Thiamin (B-1)	0.2 mg	Vitamin E	0.5 mg
Riboflavin (B-2)	0.4 mg	Calcium	169.7 mg
Niacin	1.3 mg	Iron	1.3 mg
Vitamin B-6	0.1 mg	Phosphorus	196.7 mg
Vitamin B-12	0.8 µg	Magnesium	24.7 mg
Folate (total)	48.3 µg	Zinc	1.0 mg
Vitamin C	1.2 mg	Potassium	249.2 mg

Easy Mocha Mousse

PER SERVING: 175.9 CALORIES — 3.3 g PROTEIN — 31.6 g CARBOHYDRATE — 0.6 g FIBER —
4.0 g TOTAL FAT — 3.1 g SATURATED FAT — 6.1 mg CHOLESTEROL — 423.3 mg SODIUM

2–3 teaspoons instant coffee crystals
1/4 cup hot water
1 1/4 cups 2% reduced-fat milk
1 package (3.8 ounces) instant chocolate pudding and pie filling
1 cup frozen reduced-fat whipped topping, thawed, divided

Mix coffee crystals and hot water, stirring to dissolve; stir into milk. Prepare pudding mix, using milk mixture. Fold in 3/4 cup whipped topping and spoon into dessert dishes. Garnish with remaining 1/4 cup whipped topping.

Makes 4 servings.

Nutritional Analysis per Serving

Vitamin A	43.5 RE	Vitamin D	0.8 µg
Thiamin (B-1)	.0 mg	Vitamin E	0.1 mg
Riboflavin (B-2)	0.1 mg	Calcium	98.6 mg
Niacin	0.4 mg	Iron	0.7 mg
Vitamin B-6	0.0 mg	Phosphorus	327.8 mg
Vitamin B-12	0.3 µg	Magnesium	25.5 mg
Folate (total)	4.6 µg	Zinc	0.5 mg
Vitamin C	0.8 mg	Potassium	212.8 mg

Apricot Mousse

PER SERVING: 339.0 CALORIES — 4.2 g PROTEIN — 83.3 g CARBOHYDRATE — 0.2 g FIBER —
1.9 g TOTAL FAT — 1.4 g SATURATED FAT — 0.0 mg CHOLESTEROL — 11.0 mg SODIUM

1 pound dried apricots
1 1/2 cups orange juice
1/4 cup honey
1 cup frozen reduced-fat whipped topping, thawed

Heat apricots, orange juice, and honey to boiling in medium saucepan; reduce heat and simmer, covered, until apricots are tender. Process mixture in food processor or blender until smooth. Cool. Fold whipped topping into apricot mixture; refrigerate until serving time.

Makes 6 servings.

Nutritional Analysis per Serving

Vitamin A	970.2 RE	Vitamin D	0.0 μg
Thiamin (B-1)	0.1 mg	Vitamin E	0.1 mg
Riboflavin (B-2)	0.1 mg	Calcium	53.8 mg
Niacin	3.0 mg	Iron	5.0 mg
Vitamin B-6	0.4 mg	Phosphorus	129.8 mg
Vitamin B-12	0.0 μg	Magnesium	54.7 mg
Folate (total)	21.9 μg	Zinc	0.8 mg
Vitamin C	38.3 mg	Potassium	1,529.9 mg

Apricot–Banana Mousse

PER SERVING: 131.1 CALORIES — 1.4 g PROTEIN — 24.7 g CARBOHYDRATE — 2.7 g FIBER —
3.3 g TOTAL FAT — 3.1 g SATURATED FAT — 0.0 mg CHOLESTEROL — 13.1 mg SODIUM

1 can (16 ounces) can apricot halves, drained
2 small ripe bananas
2 tablespoons lemon juice
1 cup frozen whipped topping, thawed

Process apricots, bananas, and lemon juice in food processor or blender until smooth. Fold whipped topping into fruit mixture; spoon into parfait glasses or dessert dishes. Refrigerate until chilled.

Makes 4 servings.

Nutritional Analysis per Serving

Vitamin A	210.1 RE	Vitamin D	0.0 µg
Thiamin (B-1)	0.1 mg	Vitamin E	0.2 mg
Riboflavin (B-2)	0.1 mg	Calcium	13.1 mg
Niacin	0.8 mg	Iron	0.8 mg
Vitamin B-6	0.4 mg	Phosphorus	30.4 mg
Vitamin B-12	0.0 µg	Magnesium	27.8 mg
Folate (total)	14.5 µg	Zinc	0.2 mg
Vitamin C	10.9 mg	Potassium	417.7 mg

Avocado Crème

PER SERVING: 256.4 CALORIES — 2.4 g PROTEIN — 31.9 g CARBOHYDRATE — 4.2 g FIBER —
15.2 g TOTAL FAT — 2.5 g SATURATED FAT — 2.1 mg CHOLESTEROL — 90.7 mg SODIUM

2 large, ripe avocados, peeled, pitted
$1/2$–$3/4$ cup sugar*
$1/4$ cup whole milk
$1/4$ cup fresh lime juice
$1/8$ teaspoon salt

Process all ingredients in food processor or blender until
smooth. Spoon into individual dishes and refrigerate until chilled.
Makes 4 servings.

*Can substitute 18 packets of Equal

Nutritional Analysis per Serving

Vitamin A	56.6 RE	Vitamin D	0.2 µg
Thiamin (B-1)	0.1 mg	Vitamin E	1.2 mg
Riboflavin (B-2)	0.1 mg	Calcium	29.1 mg
Niacin	1.7 mg	Iron	1.0 mg
Vitamin B-6	0.3 mg	Phosphorus	51.4 mg
Vitamin B-12	0.1 µg	Magnesium	37.7 mg
Folate (total)	58.0 µg	Zinc	0.4 mg
Vitamin C	11.3 mg	Potassium	578.1 mg

Orange Yogurt Mousse

PER SERVING: 118.2 CALORIES — 4.6 g PROTEIN — 23.3 g CARBOHYDRATE — 0.0 g FIBER —
0.9 g TOTAL FAT — 0.6 g SATURATED FAT — 3.4 mg CHOLESTEROL — 93.7 mg SODIUM

1 package (3 ounces) cherry or other fruit gelatin
1 cup boiling water
2 cups ice cubes
1 carton (8 ounces) plain low-fat yogurt
$1/2$ teaspoon vanilla

Dissolve gelatin in bowl in boiling water; add ice cubes and stir constantly until gelatin begins to thicken, 3 to 5 minutes. Remove any unmelted ice cubes. Stir in yogurt and vanilla and beat with mixer until light and fluffy. Pour into serving dishes and refrigerate until set.

Makes 4 servings.

Nutritional Analysis per Serving

Vitamin A	9.1 RE	Vitamin D	0.0 µg
Thiamin (B-1)	0.0 mg	Vitamin E	0.0 mg
Riboflavin (B-2)	0.1 mg	Calcium	104.5 mg
Niacin	0.1 mg	Iron	0.1 mg
Vitamin B-6	0.0 mg	Phosphorus	111.9 mg
Vitamin B-12	0.3 µg	Magnesium	10.1 mg
Folate (total)	6.9 µg	Zinc	0.5 mg
Vitamin C	0.5 mg	Potassium	134.9 mg

Honey Custard

PER SERVING: 241.4 CALORIES — 5.8 g PROTEIN — 45.3 g CARBOHYDRATE — 0.4 g FIBER —
2.7 g TOTAL FAT — 1.2 g SATURATED FAT — 58.0 mg CHOLESTEROL — 48.6 mg SODIUM

1 tablespoon cornstarch

$1/4$ cup honey

1 cup 2% reduced-fat milk

1 egg, beaten

2 cups cooked rice

2 tablespoons vanilla

Ground cinnamon, as garnish

Ground nutmeg, as garnish

Blend cornstarch and honey in medium saucepan until smooth; whisk in milk and heat to boiling. Whisk about $1/2$ cup milk mixture into egg; whisk egg mixture into saucepan. Stir in rice. Cook over low heat, stirring constantly, until mixture thickens, about 5 minutes.

Stir in vanilla; serve warm, or refrigerate and serve cold. Sprinkle generously with cinnamon and nutmeg.

Makes 4 servings.

Nutritional Analysis per Serving

Vitamin A	58.6 RE	Vitamin D	0.8 µg
Thiamin (B-1)	0.2 mg	Vitamin E	0.2 mg
Riboflavin (B-2)	0.2 mg	Calcium	90.4 mg
Niacin	1.3 mg	Iron	1.3 mg
Vitamin B-6	0.1 mg	Phosphorus	115.6 mg
Vitamin B-12	0.3 µg	Magnesium	20.5 mg
Folate (total)	55.2 µg	Zinc	0.8 mg
Vitamin C	0.7 mg	Potassium	157.0 mg

Rich Honey Custard

PER SERVING: 270.6 CALORIES — 6.9 g PROTEIN — 41.0 g CARBOHYDRATE — 0.1 g FIBER —
9.2 g TOTAL FAT — 4.1 g SATURATED FAT — 229.7 mg CHOLESTEROL — 68.9 mg SODIUM

4 egg yolks
1/2 cup honey
2 cups whole milk
1 tablespoon vanilla extract

Beat egg yolks in bowl until thick and lemon colored; beat in
honey. Heat milk to simmering in medium saucepan. Whisk about
half the milk into egg yolk mixture; whisk yolk mixture into
remaining milk in saucepan. Cook over low heat until thickened,
2 to 3 minutes, whisking constantly; stir in vanilla.

Pour mixture into custard cups. Place custard cups in baking
pan; pour 1-inch hot water into pan. Bake, uncovered, at 350
degrees until set and sharp knife inserted between center and
outside edge comes out clean, about 45 minutes. Remove custard
cups from water and cool; refrigerate until chilled.

Makes 4 servings.

Nutritional Analysis per Serving

Vitamin A	134.8 RE	Vitamin D	1.8 µg
Thiamin (B-1)	0.1 mg	Vitamin E	0.6 mg
Riboflavin (B-2)	0.3 mg	Calcium	170.8 mg
Niacin	0.2 mg	Iron	0.8 mg
Vitamin B-6	0.1 mg	Phosphorus	196.3 mg
Vitamin B-12	1.0 µg	Magnesium	18.6 mg
Folate (total)	31.2 µg	Zinc	1.1 mg
Vitamin C	1.3 mg	Potassium	227.5 mg

Honey-Baked Custard

PER SERVING: 120.5 CALORIES — 5.9 g PROTEIN — 15.7 g CARBOHYDRATE — 0.0 g FIBER —
4.1 g TOTAL FAT — 1.7 g SATURATED FAT — 112.8 mg CHOLESTEROL — 169.6 mg SODIUM

2 cups 2% reduced-fat milk
1/4 cup honey
1/4 teaspoon salt
3 eggs, lightly beaten

Heat milk, honey, and salt to simmering in small saucepan. Gradually whisk milk mixture into eggs; pour into 6 custard cups. Place custard cups in baking pan; fill pan with 1-inch hot water. Bake, uncovered, at 375 degrees until custards are set and sharp knife inserted halfway between center and edge of cups comes out clean, about 30 minutes. Cool. Serve warm, or refrigerate and serve cold.

Makes 6 servings.

Nutritional Analysis per Serving

Vitamin A	94.1 RE	Vitamin D	1.1 µg
Thiamin (B-1)	0 mg	Vitamin E	0.3 mg
Riboflavin (B-2)	0.3 mg	Calcium	112.4 mg
Niacin	0.1 mg	Iron	0.5 mg
Vitamin B-6	0.1 mg	Phosphorus	122.3 mg
Vitamin B-12	0.5 µg	Magnesium	14.2 mg
Folate (total)	16.1 µg	Zinc	0.6 mg
Vitamin C	0.9 mg	Potassium	162.8 mg

Vanilla-Bean Custard

PER SERVING: 308.9 CALORIES — 8.1 g PROTEIN — 46.9 g CARBOHYDRATE — 0.1 g FIBER —
11.0 g TOTAL FAT — 4.8 g SATURATED FAT — 285.0 mg CHOLESTEROL — 78.4 mg SODIUM

2¼ cups whole milk

1 whole vanilla bean

5 egg yolks

½ cup honey

3 tablespoons cornstarch

Heat the milk and vanilla bean to simmering in medium saucepan; remove from heat and discard vanilla bean. Beat egg yolks, honey, and cornstarch in bowl until well blended; gradually whisk into milk mixture. Return mixture to saucepan and cook over medium heat, whisking constantly, until thickened, 3 to 5 minutes. Strain custard into a bowl; cool, stirring occasionally. Place buttered round of waxed paper on surface of custard; refrigerate until chilled.

Makes 4 servings.

Nutritional Analysis per Serving

Vitamin A	163.7 RE	Vitamin D	2.1 µg
Thiamin (B-1)	0.1 mg	Vitamin E	0.8 mg
Riboflavin (B-2)	0.4 mg	Calcium	194.4 mg
Niacin	0.2 mg	Iron	1.0 mg
Vitamin B-6	0.1 mg	Phosphorus	231.4 mg
Vitamin B-12	1.1 µg	Magnesium	20.7 mg
Folate (total)	38.0 µg	Zinc	1.3 mg
Vitamin C	1.4 mg	Potassium	250.3 mg

Peanut–Butter Custard

PER SERVING: 216.9 CALORIES — 10.4 g PROTEIN — 23.4 g CARBOHYDRATE — 1.0 g FIBER —
10.1 g TOTAL FAT — 3.0 g SATURATED FAT — 112.4 mg CHOLESTEROL — 167.5 mg SODIUM

1$^1/_4$ cups 2% reduced-fat milk

$^1/_4$ cup reduced-fat creamy peanut butter

2 eggs, beaten

3 tablespoons honey

Whisk milk and peanut butter in bowl until smooth; whisk in eggs and honey. Pour mixture into custard cups. Stand custard cups in baking pan; add 1-inch hot water to pan. Bake, uncovered, at 325 degrees until set and sharp knife inserted halfway between center and edge comes out clean, about 30 minutes. Cool; refrigerate and serve chilled.

Makes 4 servings.

Nutritional Analysis per Serving

Vitamin A	91.2 RE	Vitamin D	1.1 µg
Thiamin (B-1)	0.1 mg	Vitamin E	1.5 mg
Riboflavin (B-2)	0.3 mg	Calcium	112.5 mg
Niacin	2.7 mg	Iron	0.8 mg
Vitamin B-6	0.1 mg	Phosphorus	184.0 mg
Vitamin B-12	0.5 µg	Magnesium	44.1 mg
Folate (total)	26.7 µg	Zinc	1.1 mg
Vitamin C	0.8 mg	Potassium	276.3 mg

Easy Chocolate Bavarian Cream

PER SERVING: 159.5 CALORIES — 4.3 g PROTEIN — 21.8 g CARBOHYDRATE — 0.5 g FIBER —
8.7 g TOTAL FAT — 8.2 g SATURATED FAT — 5.7 mg CHOLESTEROL — 24.5 mg SODIUM

2 envelopes unflavored gelatin
3/4 cup very hot water
1 package (6 ounces) reduced-fat semi-sweet chocolate morsels
1 cup whole milk
1/2 teaspoon vanilla
1 heaping cup crushed ice
6 tablespoons frozen whipped topping, thawed
Chocolate curls, as garnish

Process gelatin and hot water in food processor or blender 30 seconds; add chocolate and process 15 seconds. Add milk and vanilla and process until smooth. Add ice and process until ice melts and mixture begins to thicken, 30 to 45 seconds.

Pour into 6 dessert dishes. Refrigerate until serving time, allowing at least 15 minutes. Garnish with whipped topping and chocolate curls.

Makes 6 servings.

Nutritional Analysis per Serving

Vitamin A	12.6 RE	Vitamin D	0.4 µg
Thiamin (B-1)	0.0 mg	Vitamin E	0.0 mg
Riboflavin (B-2)	0.1 mg	Calcium	49.7 mg
Niacin	0.0 mg	Iron	0.0 mg
Vitamin B-6	0.0 mg	Phosphorus	38.8 mg
Vitamin B-12	0.1 µg	Magnesium	5.8 mg
Folate (total)	2.7 µg	Zinc	0.2 mg
Vitamin C	0.4 mg	Potassium	62.7 mg

Cinnamon-Baked Bananas

PER SERVING: 241.9 CALORIES — 6.1 g PROTEIN — 44.5 g CARBOHYDRATE — 3.0 g FIBER —
5.8 g TOTAL FAT — 1.9 g SATURATED FAT — 213.9 mg CHOLESTEROL — 45.6 mg SODIUM

4 small ripe bananas, mashed
4 egg yolks
1 cup fat-free milk
¼ cup packed light brown sugar
½ teaspoon ground cinnamon

Blend all ingredients and pour into 4 custard cups. Place cups into baking pan; pour 1-inch hot water into pan. Bake, uncovered, at 350 degrees until set, about 30 minutes. Serve warm, or refrigerate and serve chilled.

Makes 4 servings.

Nutritional Analysis per Serving

Vitamin A	143.8 RE	Vitamin D	1.2 µg
Thiamin (B-1)	0.1 mg	Vitamin E	0.9 mg
Riboflavin (B-2)	0.3 mg	Calcium	120.4 mg
Niacin	0.7 mg	Iron	1.3 mg
Vitamin B-6	0.8 mg	Phosphorus	169.7 mg
Vitamin B-12	0.7 µg	Magnesium	46.6 mg
Folate (total)	49.9 µg	Zinc	1.0 mg
Vitamin C	11.4 mg	Potassium	633.6 mg

Pots de Crème Ice Cream

PER SERVING: 207.5 CALORIES — 2.6 g PROTEIN — 22.2 g CARBOHYDRATE — 1.7 g FIBER —
13.2 g TOTAL FAT — 7.9 g SATURATED FAT — 106.3 mg CHOLESTEROL — 6.7 mg SODIUM

$^1/_2$ cup water, boiling
1 package (6 ounces) reduced-fat semi-sweet chocolate chips
3 egg yolks
$^1/_2$ carton (8 ounce-size) reduced-fat frozen whipped topping, thawed

Process boiling water and chocolate in food processor or
blender until chocolate is melted. Add egg yolks one at a time,
processing until smooth after each addition. Transfer chocolate
mixture into a mixing bowl; fold in whipped topping. Turn into a
foil-lined 9 x 5 x 3-inch loaf pan and freeze until firm. Scoop into
small balls, or cut into slices to serve.

Makes 6 servings.

Nutritional Analysis per Serving

Vitamin A	49.0 RE	Vitamin D	0.6 µg
Thiamin (B-1)	0.0 mg	Vitamin E	0.6 mg
Riboflavin (B-2)	0.1 mg	Calcium	20.4 mg
Niacin	0.1 mg	Iron	1.2 mg
Vitamin B-6	0.0 mg	Phosphorus	77.9 mg
Vitamin B-12	0.3 µg	Magnesium	33.4 mg
Folate (total)	13.0 µg	Zinc	0.7 mg
Vitamin C	0.0 mg	Potassium	111.3 mg

Maple–Pumpkin Pie

PER SERVING: 303.9 CALORIES — 5.4 g PROTEIN — 44.2 g CARBOHYDRATE — 2.3 g FIBER —
12.4 g TOTAL FAT — 5.0 g SATURATED FAT — 60.2 mg CHOLESTEROL — 312.8 mg SODIUM

1 can (16 ounces) pumpkin

1²/₃ cups whole milk

2 eggs

¹/₂ cup honey

¹/₄ cup maple syrup

1 teaspoon ground cinnamon

¹/₂ teaspoon ground ginger

¹/₄ teaspoon ground cloves

¹/₂ teaspoon salt

1 unbaked deep-dish 9-inch pie crust

1 cup frozen whipped topping, thawed

Beat all ingredients, except pie crust and whipped topping
until smooth; pour into pie crust. Bake uncovered at 425 degrees
for 15 minutes. Cover lightly with aluminum foil, reduce heat to
350 degrees, and bake until set and sharp knife inserted between
center and edge comes out clean, about 55 minutes. Cool on wire
rack. Serve warm with dollops of whipped topping.

Makes 8 servings.

Nutritional Analysis per Serving

Vitamin A	1,290.5 RE	Vitamin D	0.7 µg
Thiamin (B-1)	0.1 mg	Vitamin E	0.8 mg
Riboflavin (B-2)	0.2 mg	Calcium	95.8 mg
Niacin	1.0 mg	Iron	2.0 mg
Vitamin B-6	0.1 mg	Phosphorus	105.9 mg
Vitamin B-12	0.3 µg	Magnesium	26.4 mg
Folate (total)	30.9 µg	Zinc	1.0 mg
Vitamin C	3.1 mg	Potassium	259.3 mg

Cheddar–Pineapple Casserole

PER SERVING: 250.8 CALORIES — 4.5 g PROTEIN — 46.8 g CARBOHYDRATE — 1.1 g FIBER — 6.6 g TOTAL FAT — 3.8 g SATURATED FAT — 14.3 mg CHOLESTEROL — 176.8 mg SODIUM

1 can (20 ounces) crushed pineapple, undrained
$1/2$ cup honey
3 tablespoons flour
$1/2$–1 cup (2–4 ounces) shredded reduced-fat Cheddar cheese
2–4 tablespoons melted butter or margarine
$1/2$ cup graham cracker crumbs

Drain pineapple, reserving 3 tablespoons juice. Mix honey, flour, and reserved juice in bowl. Stir in pineapple and cheese. Spoon pineapple mixture into lightly greased 1-quart casserole. Mix butter and graham cracker crumbs and sprinkle on top. Bake, uncovered, at 350 degrees until hot through, about 30 minutes.

Makes 6 servings.

Nutritional Analysis per Serving

Vitamin A	81.5 RE	Vitamin D	0.1 µg
Thiamin (B-1)	0.1 mg	Vitamin E	0.2 mg
Riboflavin (B-2)	0.1 mg	Calcium	100.0 mg
Niacin	0.5 mg	Iron	0.7 mg
Vitamin B-6	0.1 mg	Phosphorus	12.2 mg
Vitamin B-12	0.0 µg	Magnesium	14.7 mg
Folate (total)	11.5 µg	Zinc	0.2 mg
Vitamin C	9.1 mg	Potassium	135.3 mg

Cranberry Cheese Cake

PER SERVING: 408.7 CALORIES — 7.5 g PROTEIN — 64.0 g CARBOHYDRATE — 1.1 g FIBER —
13.2 g TOTAL FAT — 7.0 g SATURATED FAT — 30.1 mg CHOLESTEROL — 295.0 mg SODIUM

1 can (15 ounces) sweetened condensed milk
1 package (8 ounces) reduced-fat cream cheese, cubed, softened
1 can (16 ounces) whole cranberry sauce
$1/3$ cup lemon juice
$1/2$ teaspoon vanilla extract
1 9-inch vanilla or graham crumb crust
$3/4$ cup frozen whipped topping, thawed

Process all ingredients, except crumb crust and whipped topping, in food processor or blender until smooth. Pour mixture into crust. Freeze until firm. Remove from freezer 10 minutes before serving. Top with whipped cream.

Makes 10 servings.

Nutritional Analysis per Serving

Vitamin A	103.3 RE	Vitamin D	0.0 µg
Thiamin (B-1)	0.1 mg	Vitamin E	0.3 mg
Riboflavin (B-2)	0.3 mg	Calcium	191.9 mg
Niacin	0.2 mg	Iron	0.4 mg
Vitamin B-6	0.0 mg	Phosphorus	174.0 mg
Vitamin B-12	0.3 µg	Magnesium	15.4 mg
Folate (total)	10.4 µg	Zinc	0.5 mg
Vitamin C	5.2 mg	Potassium	277.1 mg

Apple Cake Crisp

PER SERVING: 548.3 CALORIES — 5.7 g PROTEIN — 93.7 g CARBOHYDRATE — 1.9 g FIBER —
17.6 g TOTAL FAT — 9.8 g SATURATED FAT — 39.4 mg CHOLESTEROL — 563.6 mg SODIUM

2 cans (21 ounces each) apple or other fruit pie filling
1 box (18.25 ounces) yellow cake mix
3/4–1 cup melted butter or margarine
1 1/4 quarts fat-free, no-sugar-added ice cream

Spoon pie filling into 9 x 12-inch baking pan; sprinkle
cake mix over top of pie filling and drizzle with butter. Bake,
uncovered, at 350 degrees until browned, about 50 minutes.
Serve warm with scoops of ice cream.

Makes 10 servings.

Nutritional Analysis per Serving

Vitamin A	198.5 RE	Vitamin D	0.3 µg
Thiamin (B-1)	0.1 mg	Vitamin E	0.3 mg
Riboflavin (B-2)	0.1 mg	Calcium	169.3 mg
Niacin	0.9 mg	Iron	1.1 mg
Vitamin B-6	0 mg	Phosphorus	180.1 mg
Vitamin B-12	0.1 µg	Magnesium	7.9 mg
Folate (total)	39.9 µg	Zinc	0.2 mg
Vitamin C	1.3 mg	Potassium	91.9 mg

Pineapple–Cream Cheese Cake

PER SERVING: 359.5 CALORIES — 5.4 g PROTEIN — 61.4 g CARBOHYDRATE — 0.9 g FIBER —
9.3 g TOTAL FAT — 6.3 g SATURATED FAT — 12.1 mg CHOLESTEROL — 495.5 mg SODIUM

1 package (18.25 ounces) yellow cake mix
1 package (8 ounces) reduced-fat cream cheese, softened
2 cups 2% reduced-fat milk
1 package (3.8 ounces) instant vanilla pudding
1 can (20 ounces) crushed pineapple, drained
1 carton (12 ounces) frozen reduced-fat whipped topping, thawed

Bake yellow cake mix according to package instructions in a 9 x 13-inch pan: cool.

Beat cream cheese in large bowl until fluffy; beat in milk and pudding mix; spread mixture over cake. Spread pineapple over top of cream cheese mixture; spread with whipped topping just before serving.

Makes 12 servings.

Nutritional Analysis per Serving

Vitamin A	73.6 RE	Vitamin D	0.4 µg
Thiamin (B-1)	0.1 mg	Vitamin E	0.3 mg
Riboflavin (B-2)	0.2 mg	Calcium	146.7 mg
Niacin	0.9 mg	Iron	0.7 mg
Vitamin B-6	0.1 mg	Phosphorus	272.8 mg
Vitamin B-12	0.2 µg	Magnesium	16.6 mg
Folate (total)	39.7 µg	Zinc	0.3 mg
Vitamin C	4.9 mg	Potassium	180.8 mg

Index

Beverages

Ades and Fruit Drinks

Shakes

Soups

Vegetables

Desserts

Pudding

Sherbet

CPSIA information can be obtained
at www.ICGtesting.com
Printed in the USA
JSHW031118250821
18173JS00002B/152